Dental Hard Tissues and Bonding

G. Eliades · D.C. Watts · T. Eliades (Eds.)

G. Eliades · D. C. Watts · T. Eliades (Eds.)

Dental Hard Tissues and Bonding

Interfacial Phenomena and Related Properties

With 78 Figures and 26 Tables

Springer

George Eliades, DDS, Dr. Dent.
Department of Biomaterials
School of Dentistry
University of Athens
2 Thivon Street, Goudi, 11527 Athens, Greece

David Watts, PhD, DSc, FADM
Biomaterials Research Group
School of Dentistry
The University of Manchester
Higher Cambridge Street, Manchester M15 6FH, UK

Theodore Eliades, DDS, MS, Dr. Med., PhD, FADM
Department of Orthodontics
School of Dentistry
Aristotle University of Thessaloniki
54124 Thessaloniki, Greece

ISBN-10 3-540-23408-X Springer Verlag Berlin Heidelberg New York
ISBN-13 978-3-540-23408-1 Springer Verlag Berlin Heidelberg New York

Library of Congress Control Number: 2005927147

Springer is a part of Springer Science + Business Media

springeronline.com

Editor: Gabriele Schröder, Springer Verlag Heidelberg, Germany
Desk editor: Martina Himberger, Springer Verlag Heidelberg, Germany
Production: ProEdit GmbH, Elke Beul-Göhringer, Heidelberg, Germany
Typesetting and reproduction of the figures: AM-productions GmbH, Wiesloch, Germany
Cover design: Estudio Calamar, F. Steinen-Broo, Pau/Girona, Spain

24/3151/beu-göh – 5 4 3 2 1 0 – Printed on acid-free paper

Contents

Part I – Bonding to Enamel

1 Etched Enamel Structure and Topography: Interface with Materials

F.R. Tay, D.H. Pashley

2 Bonding of Resinous Materials on Primary Enamel

A. Kakaboura, L. Papagiannoulis

3 Bond Strength to Enamel

J.M. Powers, W.H. Tate

4 Orthodontic Bonding to Wet Enamel with Water-Insensitive and Water-Activated Orthodontic Adhesive Resins

T. Eliades, G. Eliades, N. Silikas, D.C. Watts

Part II – Bonding to Dentine

5 Bonding to Dentin: Smear Layer and the Process of Hybridization

K. Van Landuyt, J. De Munck, E. Coutinho, M. Peumans, P. Lambrecht, B. Van Meerbeek

6 In Situ Photo-Polymerisation and Polymerisation-Shrinkage Phenomena

D. Watts, N. Silikas

7 Bonding in Prosthodontics with Cements

A. El Zohairy, A.J. Feilzer

Part III – Bonding to Cementum

8 Composition and Structure of Cementum: Strategies for Bonding

D. Tziafas

List of Contributors

E. Coutinho
Department of Oral Pathology
and Maxillo-Facial Surgery
Leuven BIOMAT Research Centre
Catholic University of Leuven
Kapucijnenvoer 7
3000 Leuven, Belgium

George Eliades
Department of Biomaterials
School of Dentistry
University of Athens
2, Thivon Street, Goudi
11527 Athens, Greece

Theodore Eliades,
Department of Orthodontics
School of Dentistry
Aristotle University of Thessaloniki
54124 Thessaloniki, Greece

Ahmed El-Zohairy
Department of Dental Materials
Science, ACTA
Pv 31/Dental Materials Department
Louwesweg 1, 1066 EA Amsterdam
The Netherlands

Albert J. Feilzer
Department of Dental Materials
Science, ACTA
Pv 31/Dental Materials Department
Louwesweg 1, 1066 EA Amsterdam
The Netherlands

Afrodite Kakaboura
Department of Operative Dentistry
School of Dentistry
University of Athens
2, Thivon Street, Goudi
11527 Athens, Greece

Paul Lambrechts
Department of Oral Pathology
and Maxillo-Facial Surgery
Leuven BIOMAT Research Centre
Catholic University of Leuven
Kapucijnenvoer 7
3000 Leuven, Belgium

Jan De Munck
Department of Oral Pathology
and Maxillo-Facial Surgery
Leuven BIOMAT Research Centre
Catholic University of Leuven
Kapucijnenvoer 7
3000 Leuven, Belgium

Lisa Papagiannoulis
Department of Pediatric Dentistry
School of Dentistry
University of Athens
2, Thivon Street, Goudi
11527 Athens, Greece

David H. Pashley
Division of Physiology
Department of Oral Biology
MCG School of Dentistry
1129 15th Street
Augusta, GA 30912-1129, USA

Marleen Peumans
Department of Oral Pathology
and Maxillo-Facial Surgery
Leuven BIOMAT Research Centre
Catholic University of Leuven
Kapucijnenvoer 7
3000 Leuven, Belgium

John M. Powers
Houston Biomaterials Research Center
The University of Texas Health Science
Center at Houston Dental Branch
Suite 4.133, 6516 M.D. Anderson Blvd.
Houston, TX 77030-3402, USA

Nick Silikas,
Biomaterials Research Group
School of Dentistry
The University of Manchester
Higher Cambridge Street
Manchester, M15 6FH, UK

William H. Tate
Department of Oral Pathology
and Maxillo-Facial Surgery
Leuven BIOMAT Research Centre
Catholic University of Leuven
Kapucijnenvoer 7
3000 Leuven, Belgium

Franklin R. Tay,
Department of Paediatric Dentistry
and Orthodontics
Faculty of Dentistry
University of Hong Kong
Prince Philip Dental School
34 Hospital Road, Hong Kong, China

Dimitrios Tziafas
Department of Endodontology
School of Dentistry
Aristotle University of Thessaloniki
54124 Thessaloniki, Greece

Kirsten Van Landuyt
Department of Oral Pathology
and Maxillo-Facial Surgery
Leuven BIOMAT Research Centre
Catholic University of Leuven
Kapucijnenvoer 7
3000 Leuven, Belgium

Bart Van Meerbeek
Department of Oral Pathology
and Maxillo-Facial Surgery
Leuven BIOMAT Research Centre
Catholic University of Leuven
Kapucijnenvoer 7
3000 Leuven, Belgium

David Watts
Biomaterials Research Group
School of Dentistry
The University of Manchester
Higher Cambridge Street
Manchester M15 6FH, UK

Part I
Bonding to Enamel

Etched Enamel Structure and Topography: Interface with Materials

1

F.R. Tay, D.H. Pashley

Introduction

Experiments on bonding of acrylic resins to enamel and dentine began in the early 1950s in England with Dr. Oskar Hagger. He developed a monomer based on glycerophosphoric acid dimethacrylate that was chemically cured with sulphinic acid [1]. This was shown in a Swiss patent (no. 211116, 1951) to bond to tooth structure. His work led to the development of Sevitron, an early commercial adhesive [2, 3]. In the U.S., Dr. Michael Buonocore made the second, and more important, advance in adhesive dentistry, by demonstrating that acid etching of enamel led to improved resin–enamel bonds using Sevitron-like resin formulations [4]. His rationale for acid-etching enamel was that little adhesion was obtained on unetched enamel, which he correctly surmised lacked microscopic porosities for resin infiltration. He knew that concentrated (85 wt%) phosphoric acid was used in industry to pre-treat metal surfaces prior to painting or resin coating; thus, it was logical for him to use 85% phosphoric acid for 30 s to etch enamel, followed by water rinsing. The results of his work were very controversial at the time. Many researchers regarded Dr. Buonocore's approach as unconventional and reckless because he advocated the use of dangerous, industrial-strength acids in the oral cavity. Over the next 10 years, many investigators confirmed the utility of acid-etching enamel to increase resin–enamel bond strengths. The concentration of the phosphoric acid was subsequently reduced to 50% [5], and more recently to 32–37%. With the recognition that primary tooth enamel surfaces were largely aprismatic, etching times of 120 s were commonly used for bonding procedures for primary teeth [6]. Those etching times have been reduced to 60 s [7] and, more recently, 20–30s [8–10] for aprismatic enamel for bonding of pit and fissure sealants and orthodontic brackets.

Phosphoric acid etching worked so well for retention of pit and fissure sealants that it was natural to adopt the same acid on bur-cut enamel cavosurface margins [11]. Both a reduction in the acid concentration as well as etching time [12–14] had been proposed. Despite the availability of alternative enamel etchants such as pyruvic, citric, oxalic, nitric or maleic acid, phosphoric acid still remains the etchant of choice, with the contemporary adoption of a reduced etching time to 15 s for both prismatic and aprismatic enamel. The solutions used to etch enamel were also made into gels to permit better control of these acids, since acid etching of dentine was erroneously thought to devitalize pulps [15]. For bonding to cut enamel, it was further observed that even a 5-s etching time [16, 17], or a phos-

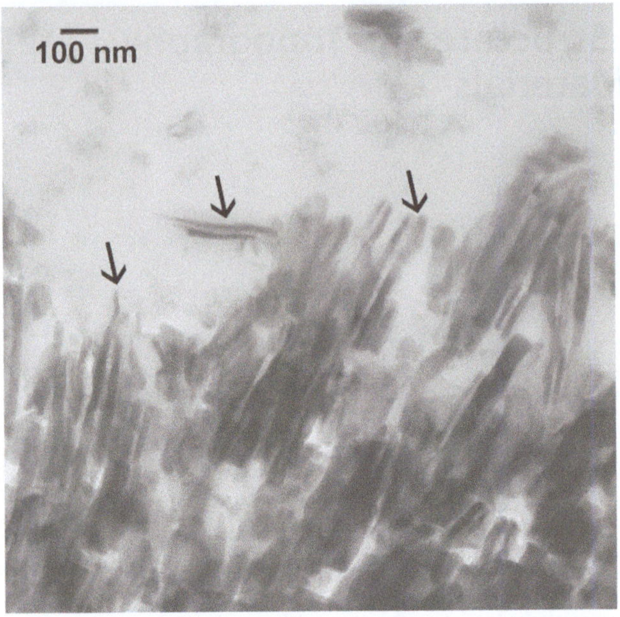

Fig. 1.1. Intra-crystallite resin encapsulation of central hole regions of partially dissolved apatites (*arrows*) in bonded enamel (unstained, undemineralized TEM)

phoric acid concentration as low as 3% [18], was sufficient to create adequate retentive patterns and bond strengths in cut enamel.

The goals of enamel etching are to clean the enamel of the surface organic pellicle in uncut enamel, to remove the enamel smear layer in cut enamel and to partially dissolve the mineral crystallites to create retentive patterns [19] for the infiltration and retention of resinous materials. There is a general consensus that acid etching increases the surface energy and lowers the contact angle of resins to enamel [20, 21]; however, there is poor correlation between the length of resin tag formation or the depth of resin penetration with the strength of resin–enamel bonds [13, 18, 22]. Etching cut enamel for 15 s, for example, has been shown to create sufficient micromechanical retention that is comparable to that achieved with 60 s of etching, without compromising microleakage along the bonded enamel interface. It has been shown that optimal enamel–resin bonds could be achieved as long as the etched enamel surface was clean and free from saliva contamination [23–25]. Increasing the length of the resin tags does not contribute substantially to the increase in cumulative surface area that is created by acid etching of cut enamel [26]. This is attributed to the ability of resin to penetrate the microporosities that are created within the partially demineralized enamel [27, 28]. A marked increase in surface area is achieved via the creation of these microporosities among the apatite crystallites, in which resin can infiltrate and result in the formation of a layer of enamel–resin composite which consists of inter- and intra-crystallite resin encapsulation (Fig. 1.1), as well as resin infiltration into the interprismatic boundaries (Fig. 1.2). First reported by Gwinnett and Matsui [29], this phenomenon of enamel hybridization parallels what was subsequently reported on dentine by Nakabayashi et al. [30].

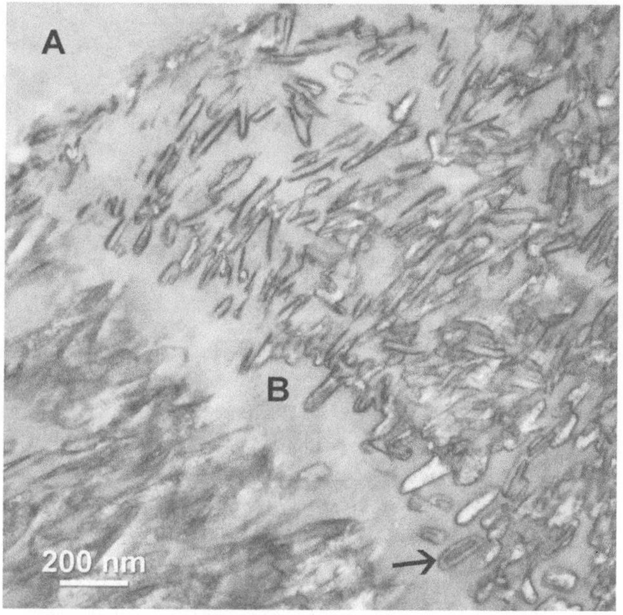

Fig. 1.2. Adhesive (*A*) infiltration into interprismatic boundaries (*B*) within enamel hybrid layer. *Arrow* indicates central hole region of a partially dissolved crystallites (stained, demineralized TEM).

With the advent of contemporary dentine adhesives that contain hydrophilic resin monomers to enhance their coupling with wet dentine substrates, there was a paradigm change by applying these adhesives simultaneously to enamel and dentine [31, 32]. Two main strategies are currently in use for bonding to enamel and dentine: the total-etch technique and the self-etch technique [33]. These adhesives are currently available as three-step, two-step and single-step systems depending on how the three cardinal steps of etching, priming and bonding to tooth substrates are accomplished or simplified [34]. Two-step systems are subdivided into the single bottle, self-priming adhesives that require a separate etching step and the self-etching primers that require an additional bonding step. The recently introduced single-step, self-etch adhesives further simplify bonding procedures into a single-step application. Both the two-step self-etching primers and the single-step (all-in-one) self-etch adhesives contain increased concentration of ionic resin monomers with acidic phosphate or carboxylic functional groups, rendering them aggressive enough to etch through the smear-layer-covered, cut dentine [35] and enamel [36]. Despite a less pronounced enamel-etching pattern, a similar retention mechanism via nanoretention of the partially dissolved apatite crystallites with resin has been observed with the use of self-etch adhesives on enamel [37]. Irrespective of how they are packaged, single-step self-etch adhesives are supplied as two-component assemblies, separating the functional acidic monomers that are liable to hydrolytic degradation from the water component which must be present to effectuate hard-tissue demineralization in order to maintain adequate shelf lives. They are mixed together immediately before use, and the mixture of hydrophilic and hydrophobic resin components is then applied to the tooth substrate. Some of the commercially available single-step, self-etch adhesives are disguised as "single-bottles" by hiding the catalysts in a sponge (AQ Bond/Touch &

Bond, Sun Medical, Shiga, Japan; Parkell, Farmington, N.Y.) or applicator tip (AQ Bond Plus/Brush&Bond, Sun Medical Inc./Parkell) which must be used for activating the adhesive [38]. No-mix, single-step self-etch adhesive is also becoming available (iBond, Heraeus Kulzer, Hanau, Germany) that can accomplish etching, priming and bonding simultaneously to enamel and dentine immediately after dispensing [39].

The Enamel Smear Layer: A Potential Problem in Bonding to Cut Enamel

During the early stages of enamel bonding, few researchers understood that bur-cut tooth surfaces were covered by the smear layer [40, 41]. These adherent layers of cutting debris masked the underlying prismatic enamel and could not be rinsed off with water (Fig. 1.3). Resins applied to smear-layer-covered surfaces bonded to the relatively weak smear layers, rather than to the underlying hard tissues. The early adhesives were relatively hydrophobic and could not penetrate these smear layers. When the bonds were stressed to failure at approximately 5 MPa, examination of both sides of the failed bonds revealed that they were covered with smear-layer material, i.e. the apparent bond strength of 5 MPa was actually a measure of the cohesive strength of smear layers [42]. Minimal or no adhesive penetration in enamel surfaces could be identified even when contemporary hydrophilic single-bottle adhesives were employed in the absence of phosphoric acid etching [43].

Morphological studies on smear layers have focused primarily on the dentine smear layer, with the intention of preserving or modifying it with dentine-adhesive primers, as these studies were performed during a period when it was consid-

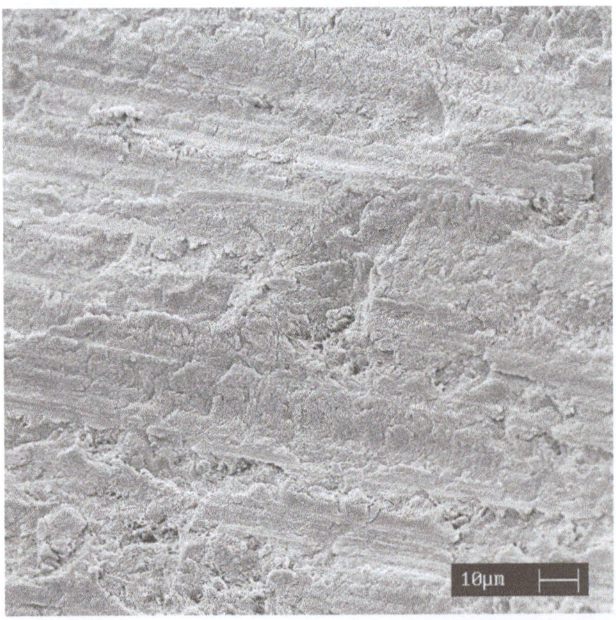

Fig. 1.3. An SEM image of the enamel smear layer after cutting enamel with a diamond bur

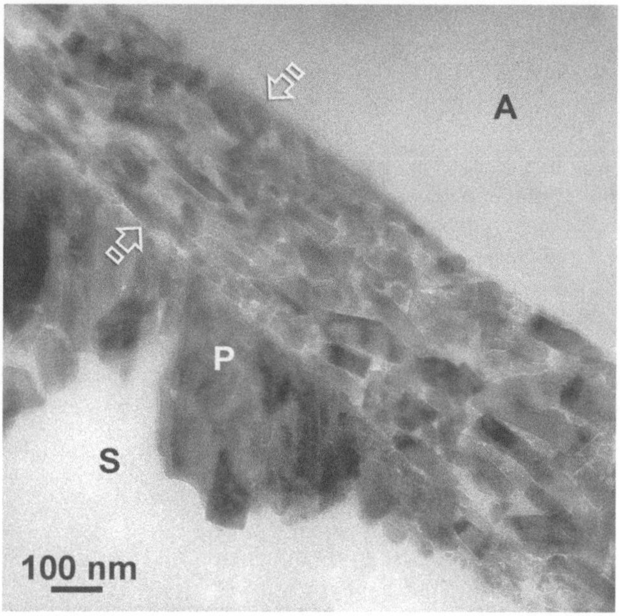

Fig. 1.4. Under TEM, the enamel smear layer (between *arrows*) appears as fractured apatite crystallites that are burnished to form a crust over the cut prismatic enamel surface (*P*). *A* adhesive, *S* space

ered a taboo to place acid directly on dentine. The preservation of the smear layers and the smear plugs within dentinal tubules was considered beneficial in reducing the hydraulic conductance in bur-cut dentine [44, 45], as dentine permeability increased rapidly during acid-etching with even 6% citric acid, reaching a maximum value as early as 15 s of etching [46]. The inclusion of bacteria in dentine smear layers also generated concerns about their rapid propagation following dissolution of the smear plugs by oral fluids that could result in their colonization within the dentinal tubules and subsequent pulpal infection [47].

Although enamel [48] and dentine smear layers [49] appear similar when examined with scanning electron microscopy, it is anticipated that considerable ultrastructural difference should exist between the two types of smear layers and should reflect the composition of the underlying hard tissue substrates from which they are derived. Despite our current knowledge on the ultrastructure of dentine smear layers, that of the enamel smear layer has not been elucidated. Dentine smear layers consisted of globular particles approximately 0.05–0.1 mm in diameter [50, 51] that were separated by water-filled channels [52]. These globular particulates probably represent fractured apatite crystallite aggregates that are burnished together by the denatured collagen remnants. Due to their higher organic content, acid etching of dentine smear layers may not result in their complete dissolution, with the possibility of entrapment of remnant minerals within the gelatinous, denatured collagen matrices [53]. A recent transmission electron microscopy (TEM) examination of the enamel smear layer by the authors showed that the latter is composed of pieces of fractured apatite crystallites that are tightly bound (e.g. by saliva glycoproteins) together to form a surface crust over the cut-enamel surface (Fig. 1.4). These fractured apatite chips are considerably larger and probably reflect the larger size of the original enamel apatite crystallites from which they are derived.

As smear layers are acid labile [54], the occurrence of an enamel smear layer did not present a challenge in bonding that involves the use of phosphoric acid etching; however, the presence of an enamel smear layer may become a potential problem when non-rinsing self-etch adhesives are used for bonding to bur-cut enamel. Similar to bonding with dentine smear layers, the less aggressive versions of self-etch adhesives must be acidic enough to etch through enamel smear layers to create micromechanical retention within the underlying prismatic enamel, with the creation of a hybridized complex [55] that consisted of a superficial hybridized enamel smear layer and a subsurface layer of hybridized prismatic enamel. For the more aggressive non-rinsing self-etch adhesives, it is likely that the enamel smear layer is completely dissolved or dispersed within the polymerized adhesive. As the inorganic content of enamel is higher than dentine, it is possible that enamel smear layers may have a higher buffering capacity for the acidic resin monomers than dentine smear layers [56]. This should be substantiated with further studies.

Application of Total-Etch Adhesives to Enamel;;

Unfilled *bis*-GMA-containing hydrophobic resins similar to those employed in pit and fissure sealants have traditionally been used for coupling of resin composites to etched enamel. Early studies in the 1970s showed that retention of resin composites to acid-etched enamel was independent of the use of an intermediate, unfilled coupling resin [57–60]. Irrespective of their viscosities, resin tags that were formed by either resin composites or unfilled hydrophobic resins into the etched-enamel prisms were all in the range of 5–10 µm. These studies were all performed in an era in which the concept of hybridization of dental hard tissues was unknown to the research community. Even at that time, Tang et al. [61] pointed out an important relation between the viscosity and adhesive penetration in etched enamel. They showed that adhesives with low viscosity produced both inter- and intraprismatic penetration in enamel after polymerization. Conversely, highly viscous adhesives result in the former type of penetration only. This difference in penetration of the adhesive in enamel was also reflected quantitatively in the tensile strengths of the resin-enamel bonds.

Several recent studies have shown that the use of a low-viscosity, unfilled resin is not necessary for effective coupling of orthodontic brackets to etched enamel [62–63]; however, only bond strengths to uncontaminated enamel were evaluated in those studies, without taking into consideration the effect of moisture contamination of the etched enamel during bracket bonding [64], or the ability of resin-sealed enamel to resist demineralization that could be induced by acidic beverages [65], or acids derived from plaque retained around brackets. It has been shown that in the absence of adjunctive fluoride treatment, significant protection against enamel demineralization may be achieved when acid-etched or hypomineralized enamel tissues were sealed with pit-and-fissure sealants, unfilled resins or dentine adhesives [66–70]. The results of these studies were also confirmed by Kuhar et al. [71]. Using electron paramagnetic resonance to monitor the diffusion of labeled molecules through acid-etched enamel, they showed that enamel permeability in both unetched bur-cut enamel and acid-etched enamel was substantially reduced with the application of a dentine adhesive such as Scotchbond Multi-Purpose Plus (3 M ESPE) to these exposed surfaces.

Bonding to Phosphoric Acid-Etched Cut Enamel;;

With the advent of the total-etch technique, it was natural to bond to etched enamel and dentine simultaneously with low-viscosity, solvented dentine adhesives that utilized hydrophilic monomers in primers. Jedrychowski et al. [72] demonstrated that a greater resistance to dislodging of resins by shear forces could be achieved when an NPG-GMA type of adhesion promoter was used on acid-etched human permanent enamel. Nakabayashi et al. [26] and Hotta et al. [73] found that in the absence of hydrophilic adhesion promoters, penetration of MMA-TBB resin into acid-etched enamel was in the range of 10 µm. The depth of resin penetration, thus, was similar to the results obtained previously with either unfilled hydrophobic resins or the use of resin composites alone. Conversely, when hydrophilic monomers, such as Phenyl-P or 4-META, were incorporated into the hydrophobic MMA-TBB resin, the depth of resin penetration increased to 16 and 23 µm, respectively. Improved resin penetration into etched enamel was also achieved when HNPM was added to TEGDMA in an orthodontic adhesive [74]. A recent study showed that enamel bond strengths achieved with the use of most total-etch single-bottle adhesives were at least equal to that of a conventional unfilled resin [75]. The use of dentine primers did not exhibit an adverse effect on long-term enamel bond strength and marginal adaptation when compared with enamel bonding resins; however, care must still be exercised when these primers are used on etched enamel that has been contaminated with saliva [76].

Most of these adhesives contain solvents that could displace residual moisture from acid-etched enamel and increasing resin penetration, allowing enamel to be bonded in the presence of moisture contamination. As the moist-bonding technique is required for bonding of most total-etch adhesives to dentine [77], it is difficult and impractical to bond to dentine and enamel simultaneously by keeping dentine moist and maintaining etched enamel dry at the same time. Recent studies have shown that while most total-etch adhesives were not affected by the presence of moisture on the etched-enamel surfaces [78–80], bonding to enamel contaminated with moisture has been poor in the absence of some of these adhesives [154]. There were also some adhesives that achieved higher bond strengths when bonding was performed on moist enamel [79, 81].

The incorporation of hydrophilic resin monomers in contemporary total-etch dentine adhesives allows optimal infiltration of the acid-etched enamel, promoting the hybridization of enamel and better inter- and intra-crystallite resin encapsulation. The hybrid layers created by these dentine adhesives on etched enamel are rendered more acid-resistant when compared with unbonded enamel. This can be readily appreciated when adhesive-infiltrated enamel was acid rinsed to bring these hybridized enamel tissues into relief prior to scanning electron microscopy (SEM) examination, or when undemineralized resin-enamel interfaces were demineralized in acids for observing the thickness of the enamel hybrid layers; however, such an acquired acid resistance should be regarded as relative, as demineralization of the resin–enamel interfaces with either EDTA or formic acid resulted in complete dissolution of the mineral phase that were trapped within the hybrid layer, and only stained enamel proteins could be identified. As these specimens were demineralized en bloc before embedding with epoxy resin, apatite crystallites that were encapsulated by the adhesive resin should be present if hy-

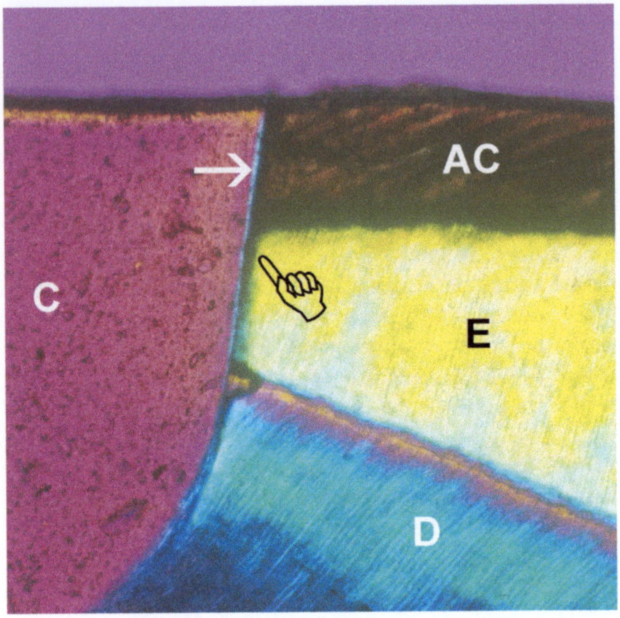

Fig. 1.5. Polarized photograph of the resin–enamel interface in Single Bond (3 M ESPE) after artificial caries challenge in the absence of adjunctive fluoride protection. A thin-wall lesion (*pointer*) extends from the superficial artificial caries zone (*AC*) into the sound enamel (*E*) beneath the cavosurface margin. *Arrow:* adhesive; *C* composite, *D* dentine

brid layers were truly impermeable. This may be partially explained by the presence of hydrophilic resin monomers in the adhesive that have an affinity for water via hydrogen bonding [82]. Although resin infiltrated, acid-etched enamel is generally thought to be more acid resistant and offers significantly better protection against subsequent demineralization when compared with unbonded enamel, the presence of these water channels within the resin-bonded enamel may account for the occasional lack of protection when adhesive-bonded cut enamel is subjected to artificial caries challenge (Fig. 1.5).

Bonding to Phosphoric Acid-Etched Uncut Enamel;;

The ability of total-etch adhesives to bond to less retentive aprismatic enamel enables aesthetic clinical procedures, such as porcelain veneers, to be performed [83]. Despite the lack of difference between bond strengths in ground and intact enamel after phosphoric acid etching [84–85], the ultrastructure of the resin–enamel interface in phosphoric acid-etched uncut enamel remains the most variable and by far the most difficult to interpret, due to the mélange of aprismatic and prismatic etching features along the same interface [86]. Much of this depends on whether the phosphoric acid is applied with or without agitation (i. e. dynamic vs static etching). This is comparable to dynamic and static priming with respect to the application of self-etching primers on enamel [87]. Generally, the surface aprismatic enamel is more resistant to etching due to the parallel arrangement of the apatite crystallites which permit a high packing density of these crystallites. There is also no interprismatic organic substance that acid can readily diffuse through to effectuate subsurface etching. Static etching results in the retention of

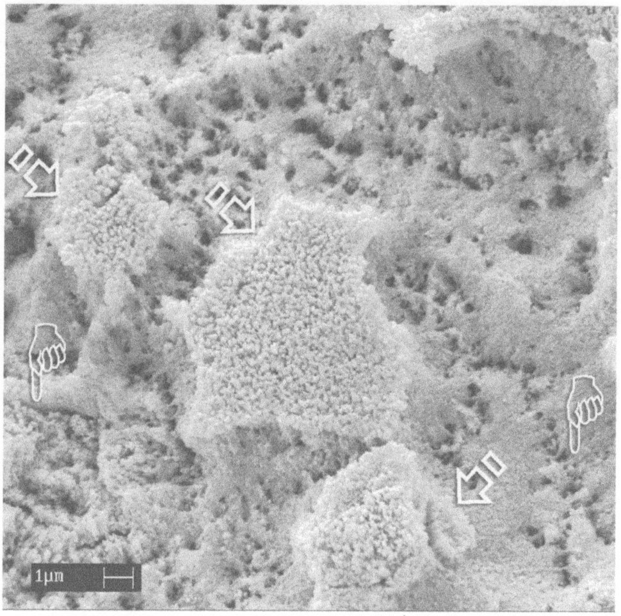

Fig. 1.6. An SEM image of uncut enamel after static application of 32% phosphoric acid for 15 s. The bulk of the aprismatic enamel is dissolved, exposing the underlying etched, porous prismatic enamel with recognizable prism boundaries (*pointers*). Remnant islands of porous aprismatic enamel are still observed (*arrows*).

the bulk of the aprismatic enamel which demonstrates a less aggressive, coral-like etching pattern that is characterized by the presence of random-occurring surface pits on the surface of the etched aprismatic enamel. Depending on the thickness of the original layer of aprismatic enamel, only sporadic islands of etched aprismatic enamel may appear on the surface (Fig. 1.6), with the underlying prismatic enamel exposed to a greater extent. Nevertheless, the increase in microporosities created along the etching front as well as the subsurface creates a high-energy surface which is optimal for resin infiltration and results in hybrid layers that are 8–10 μm thick (Fig. 1.7).

Dynamic etching brings fresh acid to the etching front, helps to dislodge loosened islands of etched enamel, and results in almost complete removal of the surface aprismatic enamel. This process exposes more of the underlying prismatic enamel that demonstrates minimal or mild etching patterns (Fig. 1.8). Even so, a high degree of variation exists between the two methods of acid application which is dependent upon the original thickness of the surface aprismatic enamel layer. It is generally understood that the formation of resin tags are minimized in phosphoric acid-etched uncut enamel, and that the predominant mode of micromechanical retention is achieved via the creation of surface and subsurface microporosities that result in an admixed zone of enamel hybridization (ca. 8–10 μm thick) consisting of both aprismatic and prismatic enamel (Fig. 1.9). Dissolution of the surface apatite crystallites results in preferential dissolution of the carbonate-rich crystallite cores (Fig. 1), forming central hole regions [88–89] that permit intra-crystallite resin infiltration [37].

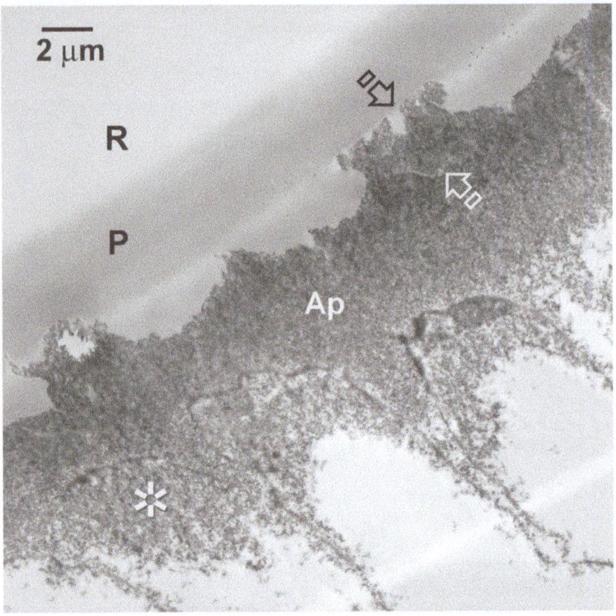

Fig. 1.7. A TEM image of the resultant hybrid layer after the application of All-Bond 2 (Bisco). Remnant islands of aprismatic enamel (between *arrows*) are seen. The enamel hybrid layer consists of both aprismatic (*Ap*) and prismatic enamel (*asterisk*). *P* primer, *R* resin

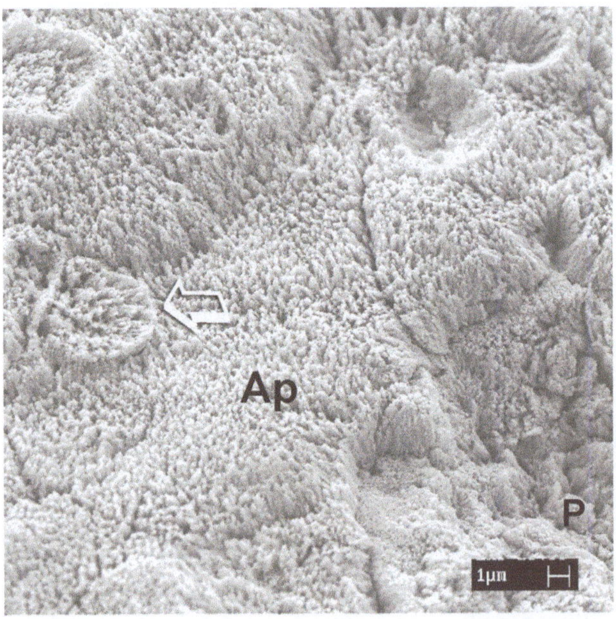

Fig. 1.8. An SEM image of uncut enamel after dynamic application of phosphoric acid. The aprismatic enamel (*Ap*) is almost completely dissolved, with partial exposure of the rod heads of the prismatic enamel (*arrow*). Complete dissolution of the aprismatic enamel on the right side reveals differentially etched enamel prisms (*P*)

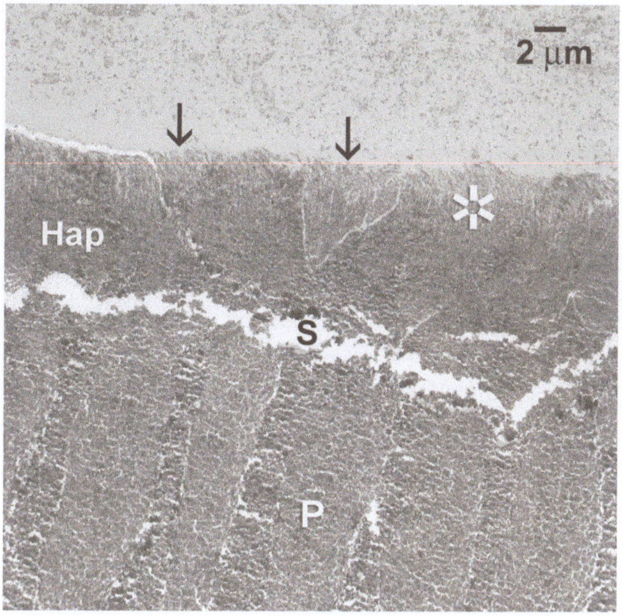

Fig. 1.9. The TEM images of the corresponding hybrid layer (*Hap*), showing the concurrent presence of aprismatic (*asterisk*) and prismatic enamel (*arrows*) along the surface of the hybrid layer. *S* space between the hybrid layer and the underlying unetched prismatic enamel (*P*)

Bonding to Primary Enamel

Due to the thicker layer of aprismatic enamel in the primary enamel [57], early recommendations for etching primary enamel called for doubling the etching time that was initially proposed for etching permanent enamel (i.e. 2 vs 1 min); however, Simonsen [7] reported that there was no difference in the retention rate of pit-and-fissure sealants when primary occlusal enamel surfaces were etched for 120 vs 60 s. Since that time, recommended etching times for permanent enamel have been reduced to 15 s. Similarly, a shorter etching time of 15 s was found to be satisfactory on intact primary enamel [25, 78]. Hosoya and Goto [90] reported that there was no difference between the appearance of prism structures by etching unground primary enamel for either 60 or 30 s. With further reduction in etching time, there was a higher incidence of the absence of prism structure after phosphoric acid etching.

The TEM micrographs of the hybrid layers in phosphoric acid-etched uncut primary enamel showed a thick layer of hybridized aprismatic enamel that was devoid of resin tags (Fig. 1.10). Conversely, resin-enamel interfaces in primary teeth with the aprismatic layer completely removed by grinding revealed the presence of resin tags and the underlying hybrid layer in prismatic enamel that is not unlike that observed in permanent enamel. No difference in bond strength-to-primary enamel was observed when different total-etch and self-etch adhesives were applied to primary enamel followed by thermocycling [91]. Similar results were reported by Shimada et al. [92]. These authors showed that, although the etching effect appeared to be more aggressive for primary enamel, there was no difference between bond strengths of primary and permanent enamel when they were bond-

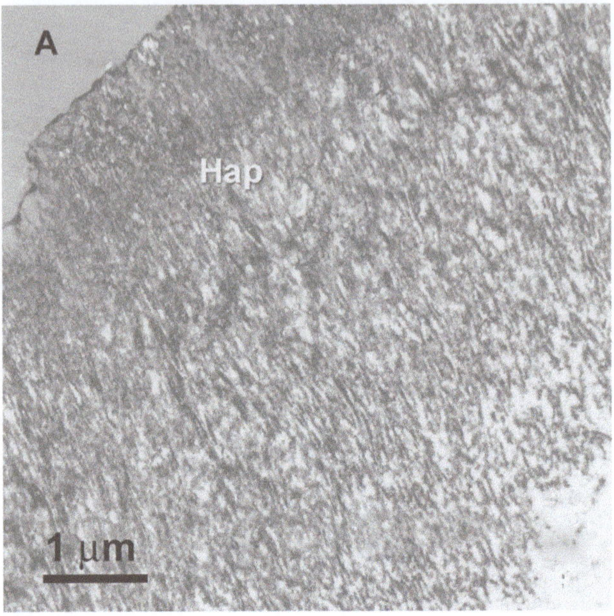

Fig. 1.10. When All-Bond 2 is applied to phosphoric acid-etched uncut primary enamel, a hybrid layer is formed exclusively in aprismatic enamel (*Hap*). This is probably due to the thicker layer of aprismatic enamel in the buccal surfaces of the primary enamel. *A* adhesive (stained, demineralized TEM)

ed using a total-etch or a self-etch adhesive, when bond strengths were assessed using the micro-shear bond strength test. Schmitt and Lee [93] also reported that there was no difference in microleakage when three-step or two-step total-etch adhesives were used in the primary or permanent dentition.

Application of Self-Etch Adhesives/Resin Cement to Enamel;;

Self-etch dentine adhesives and resin cements are becoming increasingly popular in restorative dentistry, preventive dentistry and orthodontics. With water being an integral component in these non-rinsing adhesives [35], the ambiguity in providing the optimal moisture condition for enamel and dentine bonding in the total-etch technique is eliminated [94]. Although enamel smear layers are devoid of smear plugs, post-operative sensitivity associated with the removal of the dentinal smear layer and smear plugs is also reduced when these non-rinsing adhesives are used for bonding to dentine [95]. The prospective uses of self-etch adhesives would be even more promising if they are equivalent in performance for clinical procedures such as the bonding of pit-and-fissure sealants [96] or orthodontic brackets [97–99], in which conventional phosphoric acid etching is still adopted as the mainstream technique; however, the use of self-etch adhesives is aggressively promoted by orthodontic manufacturers and is gradually gaining acceptance by clinicians, as it has been shown that a phosphoric acid concentration as low as 2% is adequate for bonding of brackets [100], with the additional benefit of preventing enamel damage when the brackets are removed at the end of treatment [101].

Aggressiveness of Self-Etch Adhesives

Unlike bonding to dentine, application of self-etch adhesives to enamel has been a controversial issue, particularly when mild self-etch adhesives are used on uncut enamel. Contemporary self-etch adhesive systems vary in their degree of aggressiveness which is dependent upon the concentration of the acidic resin monomers present, as well as the acidity (i.e. pKa) of the specific acidic monomers. This difference in aggressiveness influences the ability of self-etch adhesives to penetrate or dissolve enamel and dentine smear layers and to demineralize and bond to the subsurface bonding substrates [35]. The more aggressive versions can completely dissolve or disperse smear layers, forming thick hybrid layers in cut enamel and dentine that approach those achieved with conventional phosphoric acid etching. Conversely, the less aggressive versions incorporate smear layers as part of the bonded interface, forming only thin hybrid layers in intact dentine or enamel that are less than 1–2 μm thick. For bonding to uncut enamel, the efficacy of self-etch adhesives is dependent upon their ability to demineralize the more acid-resistant aprismatic enamel layer [36, 37]. Yoshiyama et al. [102] and Hara et al. [103] reported that bonding of self-etching adhesives to ground enamel was inferior when compared with single-bottle and multiple-step, total-etch systems which utilize phosphoric acid as a separate conditioner. Whereas some studies supported the manufacturers' recommendations that the adjunctive use of phosphoric acid etching is necessary when bonding to this substrate [37, 84], others showed that there were no differences among the bond strengths of mild self-etch and total-etch adhesives to unground enamel [85, 92, 103–105]. Although well-defined enamel etching patterns and resin tag formation are not prerequisites for achieving strong initial enamel bonds [37, 106], they have been associated with the stability [107] and improved survival rate of enamel bonds created in vivo. Although the adhesion-promoting ability of contemporary, mild self-etch adhesives may be equivalent to that of phosphoric acid-etched enamel, the thin lamina-like resin penetration produced on unground enamel with mild self-etch adhesives may not sustain cyclic stresses as favorably as deeper resin infiltration in both aprismatic and prismatic enamel that is promoted by the use of more aggressive self-etch adhesives or phosphoric acid etching [108]. A significant decline in enamel bond strengths was observed for some mild self-etching primer systems such as Imperva Fluoro Bond (Shofu), Clearfil Liner Bond II (Kuraray), and Mac Bond II (Tokuyama) after thermal cycling. Conversely, no significant decrease in enamel bond strengths was observed for some total-etch single-bottle adhesives to enamel after thermal cycling. Another important factor that influences the longevity of bonds made by mild self-etch adhesives on enamel is the ability of thin resin–enamel interfaces to resist fatigue stresses. A recent study by Nikaido et al. [109] on the bonding of Clearfil Liner Bond II to bur-cut dentine with thick smear layers reported a substantial decline in microtensile bond strength after fatigue load cycling. Similar tests should be performed in the future to evaluate the bonds made by mild self-etch adhesives to enamel.

Bonding to Cut Enamel

Studies on the bonding of self-etch adhesives to smear layer-covered dentine and enamel were traditionally performed by manufacturers on thin smear layers that were created using 600-grit silicon carbide papers; however, smear layers produced clinically are thicker but can be approximated by using 180-grit SiC paper [110]. Although contemporary self-etch adhesives have been improved considerably by increasing the concentration of acidic resin monomers in their composition [111–112], there is still the danger that they may be buffered by the mineral content of thick smear layers [56]. Recent reports have suggested that some of the less aggressive versions of self-etching primers failed to etch through clinically relevant, thick smear layers produced by diamond burs [113], resulting in decreases in tensile bond strengths after fatigue load cycling [112]. Conversely, there was no drop in dentine bond strengths in specimens that were prepared using 600-grit silicon carbide papers; however, no data are yet available on the ability of self-etch adhesives to penetrate clinically relevant, thick enamel smear layers.

In order to evaluate the ability of some of the latest two-step and single-step self-etch adhesives to dissolve thick enamel smear layers, the authors applied these adhesives to human enamel which was prepared using coarse diamond burs. After applying the adhesives according to the manufacturers' instructions, the unpolymerized adhesives were removed by rinsing the surface with acetone. Mild self-etch adhesives, such as iBond (single-step; Heraeus Kulzer); Brush&Bond (single-step; Parkell) and OptiBond Solo Plus Self-Etch System (two step; Sybron-Kerr), did not completely remove the enamel smear layer (Fig. 1.11). For these adhesives to bond efficiently to cut enamel, they must be able to diffuse through the remnant smear layer and etch into the underlying intact enamel. For Clearfil SE Bond (two

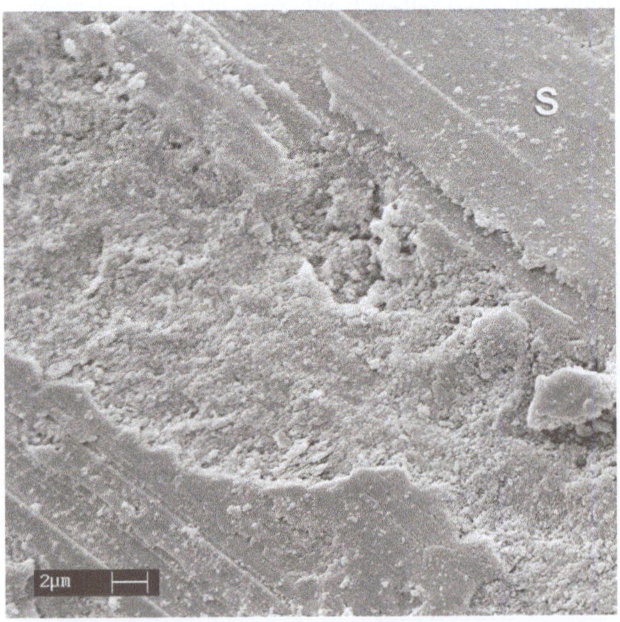

Fig. 1.11. An SEM image of the retention of the smear layer (*S*) in cut enamel that is bonded with very mild self-etch adhesives. The unpolymerized self-etched adhesive is dissolved away to reveal the etching aggressiveness

step; Kuraray) and AdheSE (two step; Ivoclar-Vivadent), the enamel smear layer was completely dissolved, exposing mildly etched enamel prisms. With Xeno III (Dentsply DeTrey), a more aggressive etching pattern with increased microporosities could be observed within the exposed enamel prisms.

The ability to completely dissolve the enamel smear layer probably provides the morphologic background to explain the favorable bond strength and microleakage results following the use of Clearfil SE Bond on cut enamel in recent studies [85, 114–116]. It is important to stress that most in vitro bond-strength studies were performed on flat tooth surfaces that are highly compliant and with minimal polymerization shrinkage stresses consequences. With the increase in cavity configuration factors associated with clinically relevant, complex cavity preparations, the ability to relieve these shrinkage stresses is restricted [117]. Recent studies have shown that the microtensile bond strengths of different adhesives were substantially reduced when testing was performed on low-compliance, bonded-cavity preparations, when they were compared with results obtained from flat bonding surfaces. It remains to be seen whether very mild self-etch adhesives that do not completely dissolve the enamel smear layer can completely diffuse through to bond to the underlying enamel, to obtain adequate bond strength to resist the effect of polymerization shrinkage stresses in complex cavity designs.

It has been reported that with the use of mild self-etch adhesives for bonding of compomers, dynamic priming resulted in higher enamel bond strengths than static priming, and the best bond strengths were obtained when the enamel was etched with phosphoric acid [87]. As some of these mild, single-step self-etch adhesives have bond strengths comparable to that of compomers [118–120], it is anticipated that their bonding to cut enamel would be enhanced with the use of dynamic priming, in a way that is comparable to the improved results achieved when these adhesives were applied with dynamic priming to dentine prepared with thick smear layer [121]. The differences in the ultrastructure of resin–enamel interfaces after static (i.e. passive application) and dynamic priming (i.e. agitated application) of one of these mild, single-step self-etch adhesive (One-Up Bond F, Tokuyama), and its application to phosphoric acid-etched cut enamel is illustrated. This glass ionomer-based self-etch adhesive contained basic fluoroaluminosilicate glass fillers that can release fluoride after polymerization; however, there is a possibility that acidic resin monomers will be buffered by the basic glass fillers if the mixed adhesive is allowed to stand for a long time prior to application. With static priming, the mixed self-etch adhesive was left on the surface of the cut enamel for 20 s without agitation, as recommended by the manufacturer. The results showed that One-Up Bond F, when applied without agitation, had a very mild etching effect that did not always etch through the enamel smear layer (Fig. 1.12). Under such a circumstance, the hybrid layer consisted only of the hybridized enamel smear layer and did not incorporate the underlying prismatic enamel. In other areas that had thinner enamel smear layers, the self-etch adhesive diffused through the smear layer and incorporated the demineralized smear layer as part of the enamel hybrid layer. A hybridized complex was formed that consisted of a surface layer of hybridized enamel smear layer and a narrow zone of hybridized enamel.

With dynamic priming, One-Up Bond F was applied to cut enamel for 20 s with continuous agitation, but without any rinsing. The enamel smear layer was com-

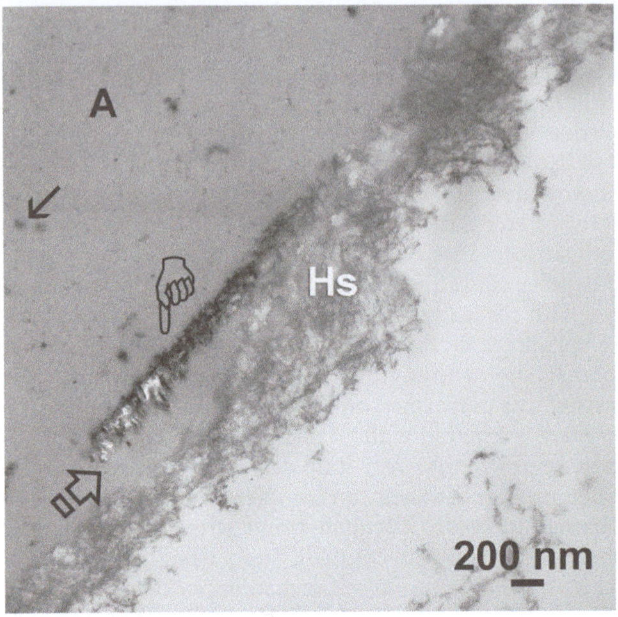

Fig. 1.12. Stained, demineralized TEM shows the static application of a mild single-step, filled, self-etch adhesive, One-Up Bond F (Tokuyama) to cut enamel. Incompletely demineralized smear-layer remnants (*pointer*) are retained within the adhesive. The hybrid layer is formed completely within the smear layer (*Hs*). *A* adhesive. *Arrow* indicates glass ionomer-type fillers

pletely dispersed and dissolved, and a 100- to 200-nm thick hybrid layer was formed that consisted exclusively of hybridized prismatic enamel. When the adhesive was applied after phosphoric acid-etching pretreatment, the enamel smear layer was also completely dissolved and rinsed away. A thicker hybrid layer was formed in areas where there was differential etching of the enamel prisms (Fig. 1.13). These results suggested that potentially weak interfaces may be created when very mild self-etch adhesives are applied to bur-cut enamel with thick smear layers, using the static application technique recommended by manufacturers. The bonding capacity created by these weak interfaces may not be sufficient to resist the polymerization shrinkage stresses that are exerted along the cavity walls of deep, complex cavities during the initial stages of restoration, and to resist long-term masticatory or parafunctional stresses.

The original claim that compomers are self-etching and do not require additional adhesive application has been shown to be largely unfounded [122–125]. With the continuous upsurge of interest in providing bonding protocols that are more user-friendly to clinicians, 3 M ESPE has recently introduced Rely-X Unicem, a self-adhesive, fluoride-releasing, dual-curable, resin composite cement that does not require the adjunctive use of dentine adhesives. The bonding of Rely-X Unicem to cut enamel using field emission-environmental scanning electron microscopy (FE-ESEM) permits the assessment of bonded specimens under wet conditions [126]. With the replacement of the original back-scattered electron detection mode (BSE) with the gaseous secondary electron mode (GSE), the quality of ESEM has substantially improved recently [127] and has immense potential in the direct assessment of marginal gaps in specimens that have not been subjected to dehydration under a high vacuum environmental of a conventional SEM. This replaces the more labor-intensive method for discerning true marginal gaps in

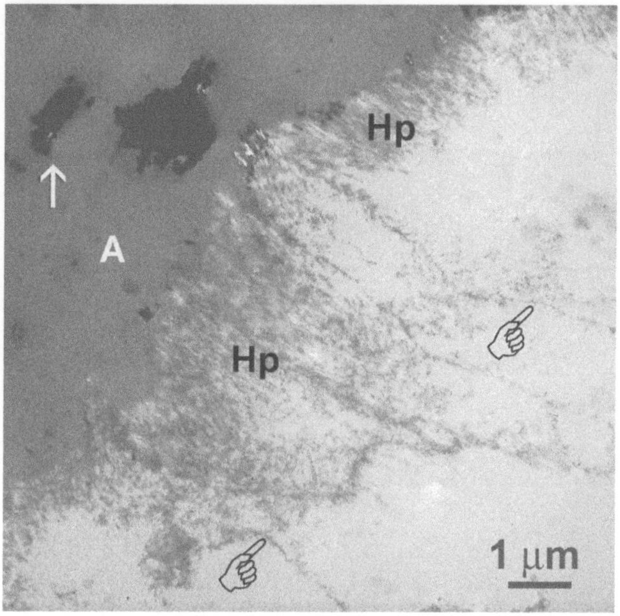

Fig. 1.13. Stained, demineralized TEM shows the application of One-Up Bond F to phosphoric acid-etched, cut enamel. Better bonding is achieved with hybrid layer formation (*Hp*) within the prismatic enamel instead of the smear layer. *Pointers* indicate prism boundaries; *arrow* indicates glass ionomer-type fillers. *A* adhesive

bonded restorations using the resin-replica technique [124]. ESEM is also useful for examining brittle dental hard tissues, such as enamel, or glass ionomer-based dental materials that are liable to crack after desiccation.

Figure 1.14 shows the resin–enamel interfaces recorded with FE-ESEM after the application of Rely-X Unicem to cut enamel in the manner that is recommended by the manufacturer (i.e. with the cement applied under some pressure). Under this condition, the self etch cement applied to a flat bonding enamel surface showed good integrity along the bonded interface, with no marginal gap formation. A thin hybrid layer that was less than 1 µm thick was also observed between the self-etch resin cement and the underlying cut enamel. Although these results are promising, further studies should be performed to assess the marginal integrity when this resin cement is used in thin layers for luting indirect restorations as well as fiber posts to root canals. The amount of curing stress generated in resin cements varies with the film thickness as well as the degree of compliance (i.e. ability to relieve shrinkage strain) of the bonding substrates [128]. In the presence of low compliance (i.e. restricted shrinkage strain), such as bonding of rigid, full coverage crowns or cast dowel cores and posts, the negative effects of polymerization shrinkage in bonded resin cements can be extreme. This is due to the very limited free surfaces around these adhesive joints that are available for flow of the setting cement to compensate for shrinkage stress development during the gel phase of polymerization [129]. Under these circumstances, the bonds formed between low-compliant adhesive joints may be spontaneously disrupted by developing shrinkage stresses [130–131].

When the thin hybrid layer of Rely-X Unicem was examined using TEM, it appeared similar to the very mild self-etch adhesives such as One-Up Bond F. The hybrid layer formed by the self-etch resin cement actually was a hybridized com-

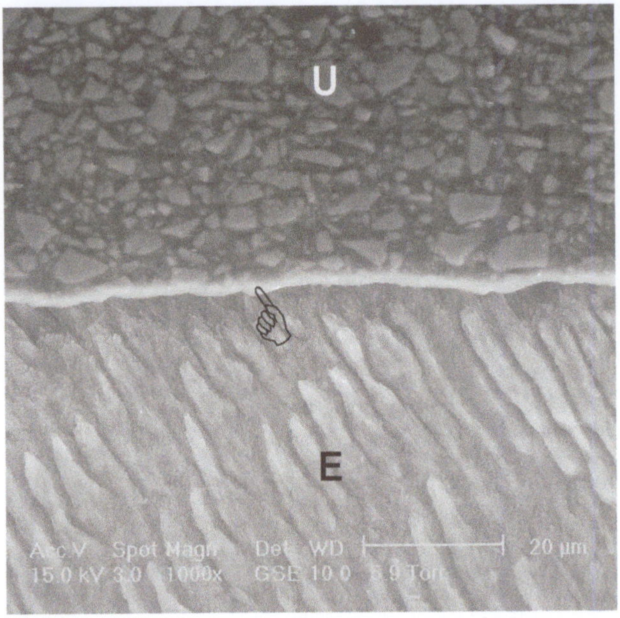

Fig. 1.14. Field emission-environmental SEM (FE-ESEM) image of the application of a self-adhesive resin cement, RelyX Unicem (3 M ESPE), to cut enamel. The integrity of the bonded interface is maintained in the absence of a low-viscosity resin or adhesive. A thin hybrid layer (*pointer*) can be seen between the resin cement (*U*) and the prismatic enamel (*E*)

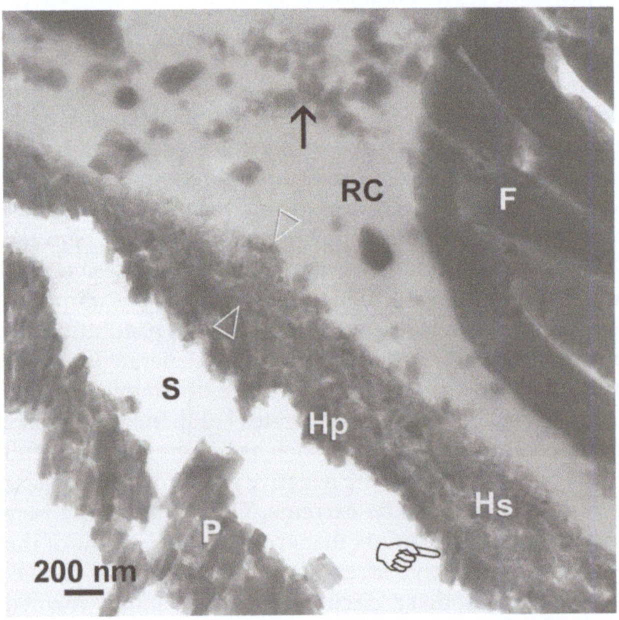

Fig. 1.15. Unstained, undemineralized TEM shows that Rely-X Unicem bonded very superficially to cut enamel. A thin, hybridized complex is formed that incorporates the enamel smear layer (*Hs*) and a single layer of enamel crystallite (*pointer*) from the prismatic enamel (*Hp*). Enamel (*P*) that is not infiltrated by the resin cement (*RC*) is fractured away, leaving empty spaces (*S*). *F* glass filler particle. *Arrow* indicates fumed silica fillers

plex that consisted partly of the surface hybridized enamel smear layer and a thin, incomplete underlying layer of hybridized prismatic enamel (Fig. 1.15). Bonding of the resin cement was limited to the hybridized enamel smear layer in some regions of the interface, where the self-etch resin cement probably did not diffuse through the original smear layer to etch the underlying enamel. This finding corresponded well with the work of De Munck et al. [132] that RelyX Unicem bonded only superficially to enamel. While the idea of bonding indirect restorations without the use of even self-etch or total-etch adhesives is certainly very attractive from the clinical perspective, further studies should be performed to investigate the use of this self-adhesive cement with the adjunctive application of mildly acidic conditioners, such as polyacrylic acid, and to compare its efficacy with glass ionomer and resin-modified glass ionomer type of luting cements to both enamel and dentine.

Bonding to Uncut Enamel

Although bonding to uncut enamel in restorative dentistry may be circumvented with the use of beveled enamel margins [133–134], such a procedure is unavoidable in the bonding of orthodontic brackets; thus, bonding to intact enamel with contemporary non-rinsing self-etch adhesives continues to be clinically relevant issue in the field of orthodontics [135–138], as the surface layer of aprismatic enamel is not removed during bracket bonding. Intact enamel is generally devoid of a smear layer; however, a surface organic pellicle may be formed on its surface that may be trapped by these non-rinsing adhesives. Also, bacteria that are present along the surface of the aprismatic enamel may also be trapped by these adhesives. The interactions of a mild, moderate and aggressive self-etch adhesive with intact enamel are represented in Figs. 16, 17 and 18, respectively.

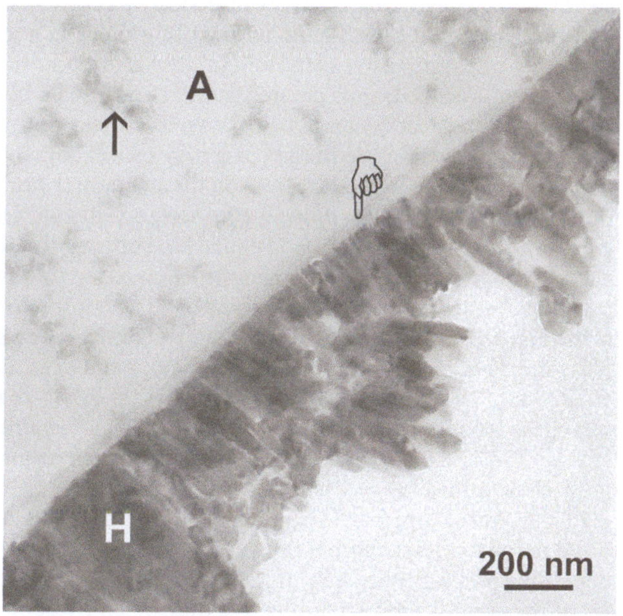

Fig. 1.16. A TEM image of the application of a mild two-step self-etch adhesive, Clearfil SE Bond (Kuraray) to uncut enamel. The hybrid layer (*H*) is very thin (200 nm) with primer infiltration around the intercrystallite spaces. The surface apatite crystallites are minimally dissolved (*pointer*). *A* adhesive; *arrow:* fumed silica

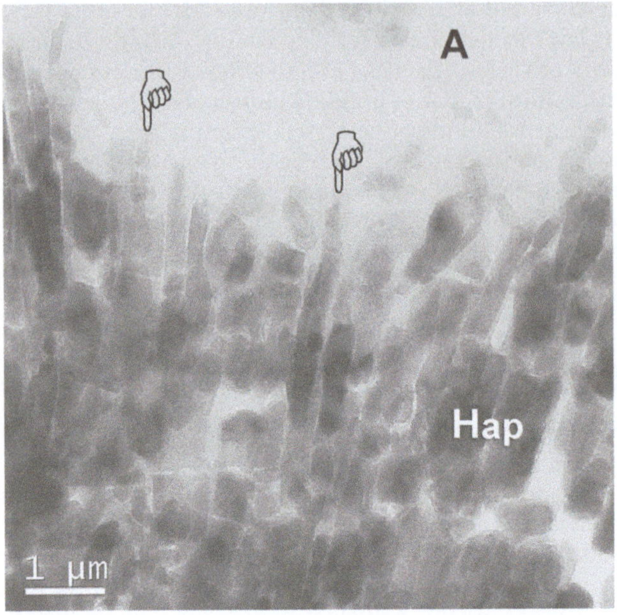

Fig. 1.17. A high-magnification TEM image of uncut enamel bonded with Xeno III (Dentsply DeTrey), a moderately aggressive one-step self-etch adhesive, showing the partially dissolved apatite crystallites (*pointers*) along the surface of the hybrid layer in aprismatic enamel (*Hap*). *A* adhesive

With the use of a mild two-step, self-etch adhesive, such as Clearfil SE Bond (Kuraray; pH=2.0), there was minimal etching of the enamel surface, with the occasional formation of shallow depressions in which apatite crystallites were exposed. The hybrid layer that was localized to aprismatic enamel was less than 200 nm thick except for regions containing the depressions, and was found to consist of a single layer or two layers of densely packed apatite crystallites that exhibited minimal dissolution (Fig. 1.16). While there is a general consensus that the moderate and aggressive self-etch adhesives are equivalent to phosphoric acid in the strengths of the bonds created in intact enamel, with the absence of any significant correlation between hybrid layer thickness and bond-strength results, the greatest controversies lie in the current research data available in the literature on the use of mild self-etch adhesives on intact enamel. For example, when Clearfil SE Bond was employed for bonding of orthodontic brackets with resin-modified glass ionomer cements, Yamada et al. [136] opined that Clearfil SE Bond exhibited no difference in shear bond strength when compared with polyacrylic acid etching; however, when this adhesive was used in conjunction with a resin composite orthodontic adhesive, it produced significantly lower shear bond strength than phosphoric acid etching. Yet, exactly the opposite results were reported by Ibarra et al. [85]. In their study, these authors showed that the microtensile bond strengths of Clearfil SE Bond to uncut bovine enamel (41.7±11.3 MPa) or cut enamel (38.6±8.8 MPa) were not significantly different from that of the use of a total-etch adhesive, Scotchbond Multi-Purpose (3M ESPE) to both uncut (37.6±9.6 MPa) and cut (44.5±6.0 MPa) enamel. It is difficult to perceive how a bond made to intact enamel can sustain fatigue loading stresses when its retention depends upon a single layer of apatite crystallite. The adhesive-promoting capacity of these mild self-etch adhesives may be equivalent to that of more aggressive

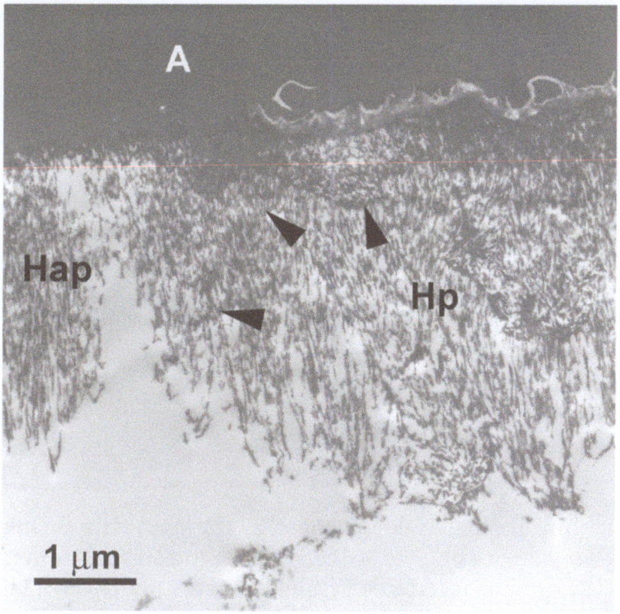

Fig. 1.18. Stained, demineralized TEM of uncut enamel bonded with Prompt L-Pop (3 M ESPE), an aggressive one-step self-etch adhesive. A 5-μm-thick hybrid layer is present, consisting of partially hybridized aprismatic enamel (*Hap*) and partially hybridized prismatic enamel (*Hp*). *Arrowheads* indicate stained interprismatic substance along the periphery of an enamel prism. *A* adhesive

systems; however, it is not until these bonds are challenged under fatigue loading that their true bonding potential is realized. Clearly, further work should be done to clarify these issues.

With the use of a moderately aggressive single-step self-etch adhesive such as Xeno III (Dentsply DeTrey; pH=1.4) on uncut enamel, the etching effect was found to be limited to the surface layer of aprismatic enamel, with the formation of a hybrid layer that was 1–1.5 μm thick. There was also evidence of external dissolution of the surface apatite crystallites (Fig. 1.17), creating more spaces for inter-crystallite resin infiltration [37]. When an aggressive single-step self-etch adhesive, such as Prompt L-Pop (3 M ESPE; pH=1.0), was applied to uncut enamel, the etching effect was comparable to that of phosphoric acid etching, with partial exposure of the underlying prismatic enamel, creating enormous microporosities for resin infiltration. The hybrid layer was about 3–5 μm thick and consisted of both hybridized aprismatic and prismatic enamel (Fig. 1.18).

Interaction of Glass Ionomer-Based Materials with Enamel

A chapter on enamel bonding would not be complete without the inclusion of the interaction of light-cured, resin-modified glass ionomer cement (RM-GIC) and auto-cured, conventional glass ionomer cement (GIC) with enamel. Compared with dentine adhesives, morphological studies on the interaction between glass ionomer-based materials with enamel are rare in the literature. This may be due to the fact that these materials, the water-based GICs in particular, are extremely sensitive to dehydration so that it is virtually impossible to examine these materials under conventional high-vacuum SEM without introducing artefactual cracks

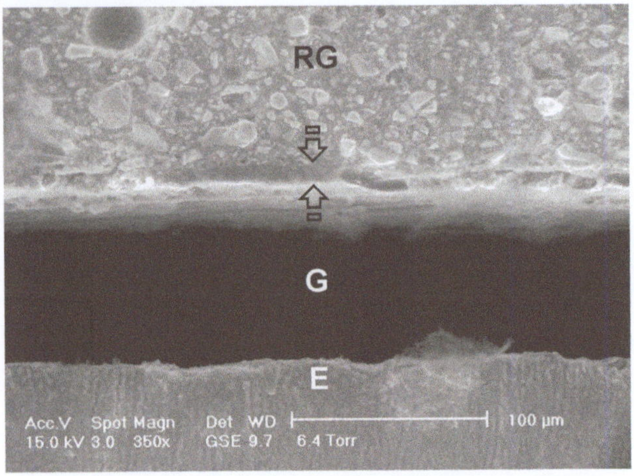

Fig. 1.19. Environmental SEM image shows the bonding of a resin-modified GIC (Fuji II LC; GC Corp.) to cut enamel without the use of a dentine conditioner. A gap (*G*) is present between the RM-GIC (*RG*) and the underlying prismatic enamel (*E*). The crust-like layer (between *arrows*), devoid of glass fillers, probably represents the interaction layer formed between the RM-GIC and the enamel smear layer

within the material. Moreover, as the materials shrink during dehydration, it is also not possible to discern artefactual gaps from true marginal gaps along GIC–enamel interfaces. While confocal microscopy [140] has enormous potential for examining the dynamic interaction along these bonded interfaces under their natural, non-dehydrated conditions, a more detailed examination of the interface between glass ionomer-based materials and bonding substrates may only be achieved with the use of cryo-SEM [141] or ESEM.

As there is a micromechanical component in the bonding mechanism of RM-GICs due to the inclusion of resinous components that can polymerize via free-radical polymerization [142], the rate and extent of the glass ionomer acid–base reaction will depend on whether these materials are light- or self-cured during the bonding procedure [143], and the subsequent water sorption that is allowed to occur [144]. The use of even short periods of conditioning with mild surface conditioners, such as 10–20% polyacrylic acid, has been shown to improve the bond strengths of RM-GICs to enamel when compared with bonding performed without pre-treatment [145]. Glasspoole et al. [48] further showed that the bond strengths of RM-GICs were significantly lower when the materials were light-cured compared with self-cured in the absence of pre-treatment.

Figures 1.19 and 1.20 are ESEM images that compared the bonding of a RM-GIC (Fuji II LC; GC Corp.) to cut enamel in the absence or presence of surface pre-treatment with polyacrylic acid. In both circumstances, an interaction layer between the RM-GIC and the enamel [141] could be identified. As the RM-GIC was light-cured immediately upon placement, these interaction layers were more likely to be created by the infiltration of resinous components of the RM-GIC into the microporosities within the enamel smear layer or conditioned enamel. Under the condition of immediate light-curing, the contribution of chemical bonding [146] via ion exchange between the GIC component and the bonding substrate [147] may not be as pronounced as when the material is allowed to set in the dark under a self-curing mode. As the specimens were examined under natural wet conditions, one can be certain that any gap observed along the resin-enamel interfaces are true gaps and not dehydration artifacts. In the case of no pre-treatment, a large

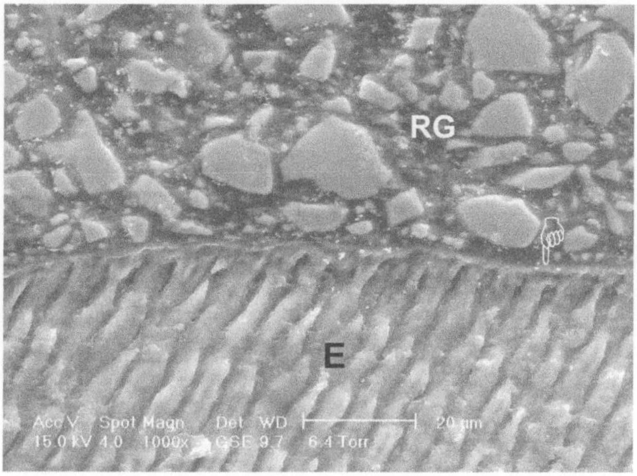

Fig. 1.20. Environmental SEM image of the bonding of Fuji II LC to cut enamel that is conditioned with 10% polyacrylic acid for 20 s. No gap occurs between the interaction layer (*pointer*) and the underlying enamel (*E*). Short resin tags are also present. *RG* RM-GIC

gap was present between the interaction layer and the underlying enamel (Fig. 1.19). It was further speculated that the interaction layer was composed largely of the resin-infiltrated smear layer, being fairly loose and slightly porous in texture. Thus, the weakest link in the interface was between this resin infiltrated smear layer (i.e. hybridized smear layer in the context of dentine adhesives) and the underlying unetched enamel. However, when enamel was first conditioned with polyacrylic acid, the smear layer could have been dissolved or dispersed, so that there was better infiltration of the resinous component of the RM-GIC into the microporosities created in the enamel. This resulted in a gap-free interface (Fig. 1.20), in which the RM-GIC was connected to the enamel via a thin interaction layer that also exhibited short resin tag formation. Several studies have shown that bonding of RM-GICs to enamel may further be improved by replacing the manufacturer-recommended surface pre-treatment protocol with 10–37% phosphoric acid [48, 148–150]. Early improvement in bond strengths of RM-GIC with light-curing and phosphoric acid etching is clinically advantageous during ligating of orthodontic brackets bonded with these materials.

There is a controversy with respect to whether the use of surface conditioners is required for conventional GICs, as their chemical bonding mechanism permits direct bonding to dental hard tissues even in the presence of a smear layer [151–152]. Attin et al. [153] showed that bond strengths of GICs to 25% polyacrylic acid-conditioned enamel did not exhibit significant improvement over unconditioned enamel. Conversely, Glasspoole et al. [48] opined that both 10% polyacrylic acid and 35% phosphoric acid improved the bond strengths of GIC to enamel, but with no difference between these two conditioning protocols. The bonding of a new ferric-oxide-containing GIC (Fuji VII; GC Corp.) to 10% polyacrylic acid-conditioned bur-cut enamel is shown in Fig. 1.21. Chemical bonding via ion exchange between the GIC and enamel also produced a thin interaction layer [141] in both cases; however, gap formation was more commonly observed when the enamel smear layer was not pre-treated with a conditioner (not shown). It is possible that ion exchange occurred only between the smear layer and the GIC, while the attachment between the smear layer and the underlying enamel remained the

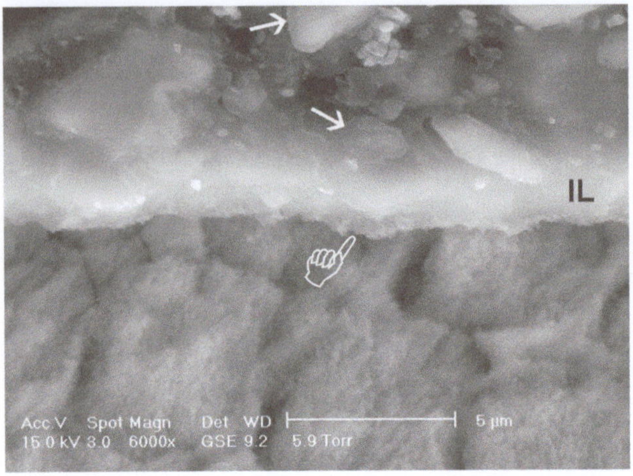

Fig. 1.21. Environmental SEM image of the bonding of a conventional GIC (Fuji VII; GC Corp.) to cut enamel. A 2-mm thick interaction layer (*IL*) is present, with the entrapment of apatite crystallites along the base of this layer (*pointer*). A siliceous hydrogel layer (*arrows*) is identified around the periphery of the ion-leachable glass fillers

weak link. When the cut enamel was pre-treated with 10% polyacrylic acid for 10 s, the smear layer could be dissolved and mild etching of the underlying enamel could be responsible for a stronger chemical union (Fig. 1.21). With the use of ESEM, the hydrated siliceous hydrogel gel layer that was formed by the leaching of ions from basic glass fillers could be clearly identified around the periphery of the glass particles. On the contrary, such a layer was not readily apparent at the SEM level in specimens bonded with the RM-GIC prior to water sorption (Fig. 20).

Conclusion

Acid etching of enamel and improvements in adhesives and resin composites have revolutionized adhesive dentistry [155]. While bonding to dentine has substantially improved over the years, the predictability of resin–dentine bonds is generally conceived to be less consistent as resin–enamel bonds. Nevertheless, there are still problems in enamel adhesion such as bonding to occlusal pits and fissures and bonding immediately to bleached enamel. The anisotropic nature of enamel also demands that the attention be paid in handling the polymerization shrinkage stresses induced by resin composite materials over enamel cavosurface margins. The recent increase in popularity of simplified-step, self-etch adhesives that are less technique sensitive, more user-friendly and simpler to use embraces new challenges in bonding to aprismatic enamel that are less frequently encountered with the use of phosphoric acid etching. The timely introduction of self-adhesive resin cement also justifies a reconsideration of a fundamental aspect in bonding to cut enamel – the enamel smear layer. Last, but not least, recent advances in the electron microscopic techniques have also facilitated studies on the bonding mechanism of glass ionomer and resin-modified glass ionomer cements to enamel.

Acknowledgements. This work was supported in part by RGC CERG grant 10204604/07840/08004/324/01, the University of Hong Kong, and grants DE014911 and DE015306 from the National Institute of Dental and Craniofacial Research.

References

1. Hagger O. New catalyst for polymerization of ethylene at room temperature. Helv Chem Acta 1948; 31:1624–1631 [in German]
2. Kramer IRH, McLean JW. Alterations in the staining reaction of dentine resulting from a constituent of a new self-polymerizing resin. Br Dent J 1952; 93:150
3. McLean JW, Kramer IRH. A clinical and pathologic evaluation of a sulfinic acid activated resin for use in restorative dentistry. Br Dent J 1952; 93:255–269
4. Buonocore MG. A simple method of increasing the adhesion of acrylic filling materials to enamel surfaces. J Dent Res 1955; 34:849–853
5. Retief DH. A comparative study of three etching solutions: effects on enamel surface and adhesive-enamel interface. J Oral Rehabil 1975; 2:75–96
6. Meola MT, Papaccio G. A scanning electron microscope study of the effect of etching time and mechanical pre-treatment on the pattern of acid etching on the enamel of primary teeth. Int Dent J 1986; 36:49–53
7. Simonsen RJ. Fissure sealants: deciduous molar retention of colored sealant with variable etch time. Quintessence Int 1978; 9:71–77
8. Eidelman E, Shapira J, Houpt M. The retention of fissure sealants using twenty-second etching time. ASDC J Dent Child 1984; 51:422–424
9. Johnston CD, Burden DJ, Hussey DL, Mitchell CA. Bonding to molars: the effect of etch time (an in vitro study). Eur J Orthod 1998; 20:195–199
10. Gardner A, Hobson R. Variations in acid-etch patterns with different acids and etch times. Am J Orthod Dentofacial Orthop 2001; 120:64–47
11. Buonocore MG, Matsui A, Gwinnett AJ. Penetration of resin dental materials into enamel surfaces with reference to bonding. Arch Oral Biol 1968; 13:61–70
12. Brännström M, Malmgren O, Nordenvall KJ. Etching of young permanent teeth with an acid gel. Am J Orthod 1982; 82:379–383
13. Legler LR, Retief DH, Bradley EL. Effects of phosphoric acid concentration and etch duration on enamel depth of etch: an in vitro study. Am J Orthod Dentofacial Orthop 1990; 98:154–160
14. Triolo PT Jr, Swift EJ Jr, Mudgil A, Levine A. Effects of etching time on enamel bond strengths. Am J Dent 1993; 6:302–304
15. Pashley DH. The effects of acid-etching on the pulpodentin complex. Oper Dent 1992; 17:229–242
16. Beech DR, Jalaly T. Bonding of polymers to enamel: influence of deposits formed during etching, etching time and period of water immersion. J Dent Res 1980; 59:1156–1162
17. Gilpatrick RO, Ross JA, Simonsen RJ. Resin-to-enamel bond strengths with various etching times. Quintessence Int 1991; 22:47–49
18. Shinchi MJ, Soma K, Nakabayashi N. The effect of phosphoric acid concentration on resin tag length and bond strength of a photo-cured resin to acid-etched enamel. Dent Mater 2000; 16:324–329
19. Silverstone LM, Saxton CA, Dogon IL, Fejerskov O. Variation in the pattern of acid etching of human dental enamel examined by scanning electron microscopy. Caries Res 1975; 9:373–387
20. Asmussen E. Penetration of restorative resins into acid etched enamel. I. Viscosity, surface tension and contact angle of restorative resin monomers. Acta Odontol Scand 1977; 35:175–182
21. Busscher HJ, Retief DH, Arends J. Relationship between surface-free energies of dental resins and bond strengths to etched enamel. Dent Mater 1987; 3:60–63
22. Uno S, Finger WJ. Effect of acid etchant composition and etch duration on enamel loss and resin composite bonding. Am J Dent 1995; 8:165–169
23. Silverstone LM, Hicks MJ, Featherstone MJ. Oral fluid contamination of etched enamel surfaces: an SEM study. J Am Dent Assoc 1985; 110:329–332
24. O'Brien JA III, Retief DH, Bradley EL, Denys FR. Effects of saliva contamination and phosphoric acid composition on bond strength. Dent Mater 1987; 3:296–302

25. Tandon S, Kumari R, Udupa S. The effect of etch-time on the bond strength of a sealant and on the etch-pattern in primary and permanent enamel: an evaluation. ASDC J Dent Child 1989; 56:186–190
26. Nakabayashi N, Takeyama M, Kojima K, Mogi M, Miura F, Masuhara E. Studies on dental self-curing resins (22) – adhesion of 4-META/MMA-TBB resin to enamel. J Jpn Soc Dent Appar Mater 1982; 23:88–92
27. Lee HL Jr. Adhesion between living tissue and plastics. I. Adhesion of epoxy and polyurethane resins to dentin and enamel. J Biomed Mater Res 1969; 3:349–367
28. Nygaard VK, Simmelink JW. Ultrastructural study of the resin infiltration zone in acid-treated human enamel. Arch Oral Biol 1978; 23:1151–1156
29. Gwinnett AJ, Matsui A. A study of enamel adhesives. The physical relationship between enamel and adhesive. Arch Oral Biol 1967; 12:1615–1620
30. Nakabayashi N, Takeyama M, Kojima K, Masuhara E. Studies on dental self-curing resins (20) – adhesion mechanism of 4-META/MMA-TBB resin to dentine. J Jpn Soc Dent Appar Mater 1982; 23:34–39
31. Fusayama T, Nakamura M, Kurosaki N, Iwaku M. Non-pressure adhesion of a new adhesive restorative resin. J Dent Res 1979; 58:1364–1370
32. Bertolotti RL. Total etch: the rational dentin bonding protocol. J Esthet Dent 1991; 3:1–6
33. Perdigão J. Dentin bonding as a function of dentin structure. Dent Clin North Am 2002; 46:277–301
34. Inoue S, Vargas MA, Abe Y, Yoshida Y, Lambrechts P, Vanherle G, Sano H, Van Meerbeek B. Microtensile bond strength of eleven contemporary adhesives to dentin. J Adhes Dent 2001; 3:237–245
35. Tay FR, Pashley DH. Aggressiveness of contemporary self-etching systems. I: Depth of penetration beyond dentin smear layers. Dent Mater 2001; 17:296–308
36. Pashley DH, Tay FR. Aggressiveness of contemporary self-etching adhesives. Part II: etching effects on unground enamel. Dent Mater 2001; 17:430–444
37. Hannig M, Bock H, Bott B, Hoth-Hannig W. Inter-crystallite nanoretention of self-etching adhesives at enamel imaged by transmission electron microscopy. Eur J Oral Sci 2002; 110:464–470
38. Tay FR, Pashley DH, Peters MC. Adhesive permeability affects composite coupling to dentin treated with a self-etch adhesive. Oper Dent 2003; 28:612–623
39. Chersoni S, Suppa P, Grandini S, Goracci C, Monticelli F, Yiu C, Huang C, Prati C, Breschi L, Ferrari M, Pashley DH, Tay FR. In vivo and in vitro permeability of one-step self-etch adhesives J Dent Res 2004; 83:459–464
40. Boyde A, Switsur VR, Steward ADG. An assessment of two new physical methods applied to the study of dental tissues. In: Hardwick JL et al. Advances in fluorine research and dental caries prevention, vol 1. Pergamon Press, Oxford, England, 1963, pp 185–193
41. Eick JD, Wilko RA, Anderson CH, Sorensen SE. Scanning electron microscopy of cut tooth surfaces and identification of debris by use of the electron microprobe. J Dent Res 1970; 49 (Suppl):1359–1368
42. Tao L, Pashley DH, Boyd L. Effect of different types of smear layers on dentin and enamel shear bond strengths. Dent Mater 1988; 4:208–216
43. Gordan VV, Vargas MA, Denehy GE. Interfacial ultrastructure of the resin–enamel region of three adhesive systems. Am J Dent 1998; 11:13–16
44. Pashley DH. Smear layer: physiological considerations. Oper Dent 1984; (Suppl 3):13–29
45. Pashley DH. Smear layer: overview of structure and function. Proc Finn Dent Soc 1992; 88 (Suppl 1):215–224
46. Pashley DH, Michelich V, Kehl T. Dentin permeability: effects of smear layer removal. J Prosthet Dent 1981; 46:531–537
47. Brännström M, Nordenvall KJ, Glantz PO. The effect of EDTA-containing surface-active solutions on the morphology of prepared dentin: an in vivo study. J Dent Res 1980; 59:1127–1131
48. Glasspoole EA, Erickson RL, Davidson CL. Effect of surface treatments on the bond strength of glass ionomers to enamel. Dent Mater 2002; 18:454–462

49. Gwinnett AJ. Smear layer: morphological considerations. Oper Dent 1984 3 (Suppl):3–12
50. Pashley DH, Tao L, Boyd L, King GE, Horner JA. Scanning electron microscopy of the substructure of smear layers in human dentine. Arch Oral Biol 1988; 33:265–270
51. Tay FR, Sano H, Carvalho R, Pashley EL, Pashley DH. An ultrastructural study of the influence of acidity of self-etching primers and smear layer thickness on bonding to intact dentin. J Adhes Dent 2000; 2:83–98
52. Pashley DH, Horner JA, Brewer PD. Interactions of conditioners on the dentin surface. Oper Dent 1992; 5 (Suppl):137–150
53. Spencer P, Wang Y, Walker MP, Swafford JR. Molecular structure of acid-etched dentin smear layers: in situ study. J Dent Res 2001; 80:1802–1807
54. Bowen RL. Adhesive bonding of various materials to hard tooth tissues: solubility of dentinal smear layer in dilute acid buffers. Int Dent J 1978; 28:97–107
55. Tay FR, Carvalho R, Sano H, Pashley DH. Effect of smear layers on the bonding of a self-etching primer to dentin. J Adhes Dent 2000; 2:99–116
56. Pahlavan A, Dennison JB, Charbeneau GT. Penetration of restorative resins into acid-etched human enamel. J Am Dent Assoc 1976: 93:1170–1176
57. Low T, Lee KW, Fraunhofer JA von. The adaptation of composite materials to etched enamel surfaces. J Oral Rehabil 1978; 5:349–355
58. Voss JE, Charbeneau GT. A scanning electron microscope comparison of three methods of bonding resin to enamel rod ends and longitudinally cut enamel. J Am Dent Assoc 1979; 98:384–389
59. ten Cate JM, Keizer S, Arends J. Polymer adhesion to enamel. The influence of viscosity and penetration. J Oral Rehabil 1977; 4:149–156
60. O'Brien KD, Watts DC, Read MJ. Light cured direct bonding: Is it necessary to use a primer? Eur J Orthod 1991; 13:22–26
61. Tang AT, Bjorkman L, Adamczak E, Andlin-Sobocki A, Ekstrand J. In vitro shear bond strength of orthodontic bondings without liquid resin. Acta Odontol Scand 2000; 58:44–48
62. Schaneveldt S, Foley TF. Bond strength comparison of moisture-insensitive primers. Am J Orthod Dentofacial Orthop 2002; 122:267–273
63. Dincer B, Hazar S, Sen BH. Scanning electron microscope study of the effects of soft drinks on etched and sealed enamel. Am J Orthod Dentofacial Orthop 2002; 122:135–141
64. Nakabayashi N, Kojima K, Masuhara E. The promotion of adhesion by the infiltration of monomers into tooth substrates. J Biomed Mater Res 1982; 16:265–273
65. Donly KJ, Ruiz M. In vitro demineralization inhibition of enamel caries utilizing an unfilled resin. Clin Prev Dent 1992; 14:22–24
66. Frazier MC, Southard TE, Doster PM. Prevention of enamel demineralization during orthodontic treatment: an in vitro study using pit and fissure sealants. Am J Orthod Dentofacial Orthop 1996; 110:459–465
67. García-Godoy F, Summitt JB, Donly KJ. Caries progression of white spot lesions sealed with an unfilled resin. J Clin Pediatr Dent 1997; 21:141–143
68. Glasspoole EA, Erickson RL, Davidson CL. Protective effects of resin impregnation on demineralization of enamel. Am J Dent 1999; 12:315–320
69. Tantbirojn D, Rozzi SM, Mitra SB, Kedrowski BL, Douglas WH. In vitro inhibition of enamel demineralization by a polymerizable amphiphilic film. Eur J Oral Sci 2000; 108:564–568
70. Gray GB, Shellis P. Infiltration of resin into white spot caries-like lesions of enamel: an in vitro study. Eur J Prosthodont Restor Dent 2002; 10:27–32
71. Kuhar M, Cevc P, Schara M, Funduk N. In vitro permeability and scanning electron microscopy study of acid-etched and ground enamel surfaces protected with dental adhesive coating. J Oral Rehabil 1999; 26:722–730
72. Jedrychowski JR, Caputo AA, Foliart R. Effects of adhesion promoters on resin-enamel retention. J Dent Res 1979; 58:1371–1376
73. Hotta K, Mogi M, Miura F, Nakabayashi N. Effect of 4-MET on bond strength and penetration of monomers into enamel. Dent Mater 1992; 8:173–175
74. Gunadi G, Nakabayashi N. Preparation of an effective light-cured bonding agent for orthodontic application. Dent Mater 1997; 13:7–12

75. Swift EJ Jr, Perdigão J, Heymann HO. Enamel bond strengths of "one-bottle" adhesives. Pediatr Dent 1998; 20:259–262
76. Frankenberger R, Kramer N, Petschelt A. Long-term effect of dentin primers on enamel bond strength and marginal adaptation. Oper Dent 2000; 25:11–19
77. Kanca J. Improved bond strength through acid etching of dentin and bonding to wet dentin surfaces. J Am Dent Assoc 1992; 123:35–43
78. Swift EJ Jr, Perdigão J, Heymann HO, Ritter AV. Shear bond strengths of one-bottle adhesives to moist enamel. J Esthet Dent 1999; 11:103–107
79. Walls AW, Lee J, McCabe JF. The bonding of composite resin to moist enamel. Br Dent J 2001; 191:148–150
80. Moll K, Gartner T, Haller B. Effect of moist bonding on composite/enamel bond strength. Am J Dent 2002; 15:85–90
81. Swift EJ Jr, Triolo PT Jr. Bond strengths of Scotchbond Multi-Purpose to moist dentin and enamel. Am J Dent 1992; 5:318–320
82. Zaikov GE, Iordanskii AL, Markin VS (1988). Diffusion of electrolytes in polymers. VSP BV (formerly VNU Science Press BV): Utrecht, The Netherlands, pp 48–70
83. Peumans M, Van Meerbeek B, Yoshida Y, Lambrechts P, Vanherle G. Porcelain veneers bonded to tooth structure: an ultra-morphological FE-SEM examination of the adhesive interface. Dent Mater 1999; 15:105–119
84. Kanemura N, Sano H, Tagami J. Tensile bond strength to and SEM evaluation of ground and intact enamel surfaces. J Dent 1999; 27:523–530
85. Ibarra G, Vargas MA, Armstrong SR, Cobb DS. Microtensile bond strength of self-etching adhesives to ground and unground enamel. J Adhes Dent 2002; 4:115–124
86. Kodaka T, Mori R, Miyakawa M. Sequential observations followed by acid etching on the enamel surfaces of human teeth under scanning electron microscopy at low vacuum. Microsc Res Tech 1993; 24:429–436
87. Glasspoole EA, Erickson RL, Davidson CL. Effect of enamel pretreatments on bond strength of compomer. Dent Mater 2001; 17:402–408
88. Jongebloed WL, Molenaar I, Arends J. Morphology and size-distribution of sound and acid-treated enamel crystallites. Calcif Tissue Res 1975; 19:109–123
89. Daculsi G, LeGeros RZ, Mitre D. Crystal dissolution of biological and ceramic apatites. Calcif Tissue Int 1989; 45:95–103
90. Hosoya Y, Goto G. Effects of cleaning, polishing pretreatments and acid etching times on unground primary enamel. J Pedod 1990; 14:84–92
91. Hosoya Y, Tominaga A. A comparison of five adhesive systems to primary enamel. Pediatr Dent 1999; 21:46–52
92. Shimada Y, Senawongse P, Harnirattisai C, Burrow MF, Nakaoki Y, Tagami J. Bond strength of two adhesive systems to primary and permanent enamel. Oper Dent 2002; 27:403–409
93. Schmitt DC, Lee J. Microleakage of adhesive resin systems in the primary and permanent dentitions. Pediatr Dent 2002; 24:587–593
94. Pioch T, Staehle HJ, Wurst M, Duschner H, Dörfer C. The nanoleakage phenomenon: influence of moist vs dry bonding. J Adhes Dent 2002; 4:23–30
95. Brunton PA, Cowan AJ, Wilson MA, Wilson NH. A three-year evaluation of restorations placed with a smear-layer-mediated dentin bonding agent in non-carious cervical lesions. J Adhes Dent 1999; 1:333–341
96. Gillet D, Nancy J, Dupuis V, Dorignac G. Microleakage and penetration depth of three types of materials in fissure sealant: self-etching primer vs etching: an in vitro study. J Clin Pediatr Dent 2002; 26:175–178
97. Bishara SE, VonWald L, Laffoon JF, Warren JJ. Effect of a self-etch primer/adhesive on the shear bond strength of orthodontic brackets. Am J Orthod Dentofacial Orthop 2001; 119:621–624
98. Korbmacher H, Klocke A, Huck L, Kahl-Nieke B. Enamel conditioning for orthodontic bonding with a single-step bonding agent. J Orofac Orthop 2002; 63;463–471
99. Velo S, Carano A, Carano A. Self-etching vs traditional bonding systems in orthodontics: an in vitro study. Orthod Craniofac Res 2002; 5:166–169

100. Carstensen W. Effect of reduction of phosphoric acid concentration on the shear bond strength of brackets. Am J Orthod Dentofacial Orthop 1995; 108: 274–277
101. Yoshiyama M, Matsuo T, Ebisu S, Pashley DH. Regional bond strengths of self-etching/self-priming adhesive systems. J Dent 1998; 26:609–616
102. Hara AT, Amaral CM, Pimenta LA, Sinhoreti MA. Shear bond strength of hydrophilic adhesive systems to enamel. Am J Dent 1999; 12:181–184
103. Hannig M, Reinhardt KJ, Bott B. Self-etching primer vs phosphoric acid: an alternative concept for composite-to-enamel bonding. Oper Dent 1999; 24:172–180
104. Fritz UB, Diedrich P, Finger WJ. Self-etching primers: an alternative to the conventional acid etch technique? J Orofac Orthop 2001; 62:238–245
105. Hayakawa T, Nemoto K. Efficacy of self-etching primers in the adhesion of 4-META/MMA-TBB resin cement to enamel. J Adhes Dent 2002; 4:105–113
106. Perdigão J, Lopes L, Lambrechts P, Leitao J, Van Meerbeek B, Vanherle G. Effects of a self-etching primer on enamel shear bond strengths and SEM morphology. Am J Dent 1997; 10:141–146
107. Miyazaki M, Sato M, Onose H. Durability of enamel bond strength of simplified bonding systems. Oper Dent 2000; 25:75–80
108. Torii Y, Itou K, Hikasa R, Iwata S, Nishitani Y. Enamel tensile bond strength and morphology of resin-enamel interface created by acid etching system with or without moisture and self-etching priming system. J Oral Rehabil 2002; 29:528–533
109. Nikaido T, Kunzelmann KH, Chen H, Ogata M, Harada N, Yamaguchi S, Cox CF, Hickel R, Tagami J. Evaluation of thermal cycling and mechanical loading on bond strength of a self-etching primer system to dentin. Dent Mater 2002; 18:269–275
110. Koibuchi H, Yasuda N, Nakabayashi N. Bonding to dentin with a self-etching primer: the effect of smear layers. Dent Mater 2001; 17:122–126
111. Nakabayashi N, Saimi Y. Bonding to intact dentin. J Dent Res 1996; 75:1706–1715
112. Hayakawa T, Kikutake K, Nemoto K. Influence of self-etching primer treatment on the adhesion of resin composite to polished dentin and enamel. Dent Mater 1998; 14:99–105
113. Ogata M, Harada N, Yamaguchi S, Nakajima M, Tagami J. Effect of self-etching primer vs phosphoric acid etchant on bonding to bur-prepared dentin. Oper Dent 2002; 27:447–454
114. Cardoso PE, Placido E, Moura SK. Microleakage of four simplified adhesive systems under thermal and mechanical stresses. Am J Dent 2002; 15:164–168
115. Kaaden C, Powers JM, Friedl KH, Schmalz G. Bond strength of self-etching adhesives to dental hard tissues. Clin Oral Investig 2002; 6:155–160
116. Shimada Y, Tagami J. Effects of regional enamel and prism orientation on resin bonding. Oper Dent 2003; 28:20–27
117. Davidson CL, de Gee AJ, Feilzer A. The competition between the composite–dentin bond strength and the polymerization contraction stress. J Dent Res 1984; 63:1396–1399
118. Yoshikawa T, Sano H, Burrow MF, Tagami J, Pashley DH. Effects of dentin depth and cavity configuration on bond strength. J Dent Res 1999; 78:898–905
119. Miyazaki S, Iwasaki K, Onose H, Moore BK. Enamel and dentin bond strengths of single application bonding systems. Am J Dent 2001; 14:363–366
120. Miyazaki M, Iwasaki K, Onose H. Adhesion of single application bonding systems to bovine enamel and dentin. Oper Dent 2002; 27:88–94
121. Chan KM, Tay FR, King NM, Imazato S, Pashley DH. Effects of agitation of self-etching primers/adhesives on resin–dentin bond strength. Am J Dent 2003; 16:340–346
122. Kugel G, Perry RD, Hoang E, Hoang T, Ferrari M. Dyract compomer: comparison of total etch vs no etch technique. Gen Dent 1998; 46:604–606
123. Manhart J, Chen HY, Kunzelmann KH, Hickel R. Bond strength of a compomer to dentin under various surface conditions. Clin Oral Investig 1999; 3:175–180
124. Luo Y, Tay FR, Lo EC, Wei SH. Marginal adaptation of a new compomer under different conditioning methods. J Dent 2000; 28:495–500
125. Tate WH, You C, Powers JM. Bond strength of compomers to human enamel. Oper Dent 2000; 25:283–291

126. Goracci C, Ferrari M, Grandini S, Monticelli F, Tay FR. Bonding of a self-adhesive resin cement to dental hard tissues. J Adhes Dent (in press)
127. Cowan AJ, Wilson NH, Wilson MA, Watts DC. The application of ESEM in dental materials research. J Dent 1996; 24:375–377
128. Alster D, Venhoven BA, Feilzer AJ, Davidson CL. Influence of compliance of the substrate materials on polymerization contraction stress in thin resin composite layers. Biomaterials 1997; 18:337–341
129. Feilzer AJ, De Gee AJ, Davidson CL. Increased wall-to-wall curing contraction in thin bonded resin layers. J Dent Res 1989; 68:48–50
130. Davidson CL, Van Zeghbroeck L, Feilzer AJ. Destructive stresses in adhesive luting cements. J Dent Res 1991; 70:880–882
131. Verzijden CW, Feilzer AJ, Creugers NH, Davidson CL. The influence of polymerization shrinkage of resin cements on bonding to metal. J Dent Res 1992; 71:410–413
132. De Munck J, Vargas M, Van Landuyt K, Hikita K, Lambrechts P, Van Meerbeek B. Bonding of an auto-adhesive luting material to enamel and dentin. Dent Mater 2004; 20:963–971
133. Opdam NJ, Roeters JJ, Kuijs R, Burgersdijk RC. Necessity of bevels for box only class II composite restorations. J Prosthet Dent 1998; 80:274–279
134. Hoelscher DC, Gregory WA, Linger JB, Pink FE. Effect of light source position and bevel placement on facial margin adaptation of resin-based composite restorations. Am J Dent 2000; 13:171–175
135. Arnold RW, Combe EC, Warford JH Jr. Bonding of stainless steel brackets to enamel with a new self-etching primer. Am J Orthod Dentofacial Orthop 2002; 122: 274–276
136. Yamada R, Hayakawa T, Kasai K. Effect of using self-etching primer for bonding orthodontic brackets. Angle Orthod 2002; 558–564
137. Bishara SE, Ajlouni R, Laffoon JF, Warren JJ. Effect of a fluoride-releasing self-etch acidic primer on the shear bond strength of orthodontic brackets. Angle Orthod 2002; 72:199–202
138. Bishara SE, Oonsombat C, Ajlouni R, Denehy G. The effect of saliva contamination on shear bond strength of orthodontic brackets when using a self-etch primer. Angle Orthod 2002; 72:554–557
139. Tay FR, Lai CNS, Chersoni S, Pashley DH, Mak YF, Suppa P, Prati C, King NM. Osmotic blistering in enamel bonded with one-step self-etch adhesives. J Dent Res 2004; 83:296–301
140. Watson TF, Pagliari D, Sidhu SK, Naasan MA. Confocal microscopic observation of structural changes in glass-ionomer cements and tooth interfaces. Biomaterials 1998; 19:581–588
141. Ngo H, Mount GJ, Peters MC. A study of glass-ionomer cement and its interface with enamel and dentin using a low-temperature, high-resolution scanning electron microscopic technique. Quintessence Int 1997; 28:63–69
142. Sidhu SK, Sherriff M, Watson TF. The effects of maturity and dehydration shrinkage on resin-modified glass-ionomer restorations. J Dent Res 1997; 76:1495–1501
143. Kakaboura A, Eliades G, Palaghias G. An FTIR study on the setting mechanism of resin-modified glass ionomer restoratives. Dent Mater 1996; 12:173–178
144. Small IC, Watson TF, Chadwick AV, Sidhu SK. Water sorption in resin-modified glass-ionomer cements: an in vitro comparison with other materials. Biomaterials 1998; 19:545–550
145. Gordan VV. Effect of conditioning times on resin-modified glass-ionomer bonding. Am J Dent 2000; 13:13–16
146. Yoshida Y, Van Meerbeek B, Nakayama Y, Snauwaert J, Hellemans L, Lambrechts P, Vanherle G, Wakasa K. Evidence of chemical bonding at biomaterial–hard tissue interfaces. J Dent Res 2000; 79:709–714
147. Sennou HE, Lebugle AA, Grégoire GL. X-ray photoelectron spectroscopy study of the dentin-glass ionomer cement interface. Dent Mater 1999; 15:229–237
148. Cortes O, García-Godoy F, Boj JR. Bond strength of resin-reinforced glass ionomer cements after enamel etching. Am J Dent 1993; 6:299–301
149. Desai M, Tyas MJ. Adhesion to enamel of light-cured poly-acid dental materials. Aust Dent J 1996; 41:393–397

150. Bishara SE, Vonwald L, Laffoon JF, Jakobsen JR. Effect of altering the type of enamel conditioner on the shear bond strength of a resin-reinforced glass ionomer adhesive. Am J Orthod Dentofacial Orthop 2000; 118:288–294
151. Arweiler NB, Auschill TM, Reich E. Does pretreatment of cavities effectively promote good marginal adaptation of glass-ionomer cements? J Adhes Dent 2000; 2:289–295
152. Tanumiharja M, Burrow MF, Cimmino A, Tyas MJ. The evaluation of four conditioners for glass ionomer cements using field-emission scanning electron microscopy. J Dent 2001; 29:131–138
153. Attin T, Buchalla W, Hellwig E. Influence of enamel conditioning on bond strength of resin-modified glass ionomer restorative materials and polyacid-modified composites. J Prosthet Dent 1996; 76:29–33
154. Jain P, Stewart GP. Effect of dentin primer on shear bond strength of composite resin to moist and dry enamel. Oper Dent 2000; 25:51–58
155. Van Meerbeek B, De Munck J, Yoshida Y, Inoue S, Vargas M, Vijay P, Van Landuyt K, Lambrechts P, Vanherle G. Buonocore memorial lecture. Adhesion to enamel and dentin: current status and future challenges. Oper Dent 2003; 28:215–235

Bonding of Resinous Materials on Primary Enamel

2

A. Kakaboura, L. Papagiannoulis

Introduction

Resin sealants are accepted as an effective procedure for controlling fissure decay in primary and permanent teeth. At the same time, increased use has been reported in resin composite restoratives in posterior teeth as substitute for amalgam.

Enamel acid etching is considered the most appropriate surface treatment to ensure retention of the resinous materials both on primary and permanent enamel. From the research point of view, very few studies evaluate the bonding of resinous materials on primary enamel. The parameters attributed to the bonding are usually assigned on tissues of permanent teeth and the results are merely extrapolated to primary analogues.

However, chemical, physiological and micromorphological differences between primary and permanent enamel have been well established. Therefore, although bonding on primary enamel may follow the principles of adhesion of resinous materials on the hard dental tissues, the individual features of the deciduous enamel make necessary the study of the subject as a separate issue.

The necessity of enamel cleaning prior to the bonding, the influence of various acid treatments on regions of the primary enamel, the bonding efficiency of resinous materials on enamel through adhesive systems and clinical data related to the retention rates of the materials are described in the present chapter.

Primary Enamel

In primary teeth the coronal part is covered by a thin enamel layer which is generally less mineralized than permanent enamel [1]. In this respect, the area of the organic/inorganic interface is greater in deciduous enamel, which contains more exogenous organic material [2]. The reduced time available for enamel maturation may account for the relatively lower mineral levels.

As in the permanent enamel, the mineralization level of the deciduous enamel is characterized by the gradient from the inside to outside, albeit with a smaller relative increase [1]. A neonatal distinct line is also obvious in the primary enamel which divides the less and the more hypomineralized enamel formed before and after birth, respectively.

As a consequence of the features described, the permeability of the deciduous is higher than that of the permanent enamel [1]; the latter also suggests higher porosity of the primary enamel, which leads to higher pore volume [2]. The thinner enamel layer, in combination with the less mineral content and the pronounced porosity, accounts for the whitish, opaque appearance of the primary enamel.

Although enamel of deciduous and permanent teeth has overall similar chemical composition, variations in carbonates have been indicated [3, 4]. Carbonate substitutions in the hydroxyapatite crystals is known to change the surface charge and the solubility of the enamel surface [5, 6].

The enamel surface itself, in both permanent and deciduous teeth, is a micromorphologically and chemically complex region; however, the deciduous enamel is considered the most variable enamel [7]. The presence of prismless (aprismatic) enamel in different areas of the same tooth [8, 9], with varying thickness (5–60 μm) [10], is the most commonly found feature in the primary enamel, although prismless enamel is also discerned in pit, fissure and cervical regions of the permanent teeth. There are significant differences in the micromorphological appearance of the prismless enamel between the permanent and primary teeth. A laminated band is found in primary prismless enamel, whereas a scale-like shape is observed in permanent teeth [11]. Many authors have reported that the primary teeth have a more pronounced layer of prismless enamel than that found on the permanent teeth [12–14]. Smooth prismless enamel in various external regions, with round depressions of unpredictable depth, has been detected in non-erupted canines and incisors [15, 16].

Regional differences have been determined in the prismless enamel. Although Whittaker [13] suggested that the outer enamel often shows prismless features, such a finding is uncommon for the area of occlusal pit-and-fissure enamel [17] and also for the one close to the top of the cusps [10]. Unlike the occlusal surface, a relative thick layer of prismless enamel mostly laminates the labial and facial surfaces, in the form of isolated islands or a continuous band [10, 18].

The crystal orientation in prismless enamel is different from that of prismatic enamel [9, 19]. In aprismatic enamel, the crystallites are arranged uni-directionally, parallel to one another with a relatively higher density and their C-axes perpendicular to the enamel [11, 12, 14, 18]. On the contrary, the prismatic enamel exhibits change of orientation within each prism; hence, the prismless enamel is presented under polarized microscopy by a uniform, homogeneous extinction of surface layer.

The structural, histological and chemical differences mentioned between primary and permanent enamel may cause differences in the etching capacity, the bonding mechanism induced and the bonding efficiency of the resinous materials.

Enamel Cleaning

Generally, organic deposits cover the enamel surfaces such as surface cuticle and stained pellicle [20]. Investigators have discovered that these remnants might interfere with the etching process, resulting in subsequent lower resin adhesion [21–24]. Enamel cleaning prior to the etching is recommended to achieve a favourable bonding surface. Since sealant placement is performed on uncut enamel areas, the removal of remnants is a necessary procedure.

Two different procedures have been introduced for primary enamel cleaning; the first consists of removing only the deposits by cleaning/polishing of the enamel, and the second of slight grinding leading to superficial enamel removal.

Controversial aspects have been drawn regarding the efficiency of the various methods suggested for facilitating the cleaning of the enamel surface [25, 26]. It is likely that after polishing with a rotating brush alone, only organic films remain on the surface [22]. Prophy pastes with fine particles result in an efficient debris and organics removal while keeping the enamel intact [25–27]. On the other hand, the respective pastes with coarse grinding particles abrade the enamel surface.

Historically, the prophy pastes with fluoride components have been avoided because fluoride was believed to provide a more resistant to acid-etching enamel surface; however, numerous studies have shown that cleaning with fluoridated prophy paste creates no negative effect on shear bond strength compared with non-fluoride media [28, 29]. On the other hand, precipitates on the enamel surfaces which are cleaned with fluoridated prophy paste should be taken into careful consideration, because it is possible to influence the longevity of the bond [25].

Pumice slurry causes especially deep scratch marks and renders adequate enamel cleaning impossible [26]. Air-polishing, used particularly for occlusal fissure cleaning, is considered an appropriate method when a prolonged (>30 s) water-washing time is followed [25]. Well-performed resin tags and higher bond strength have been achieved on air-polished pretreated, as compared with pumice-cleaned, enamel surfaces.

Grinding of the enamel surface with fine-grain diamond [18] or sandblast discs [30] causes removal of the outermost prismless enamel layer, resulting in enamel prism exposure and in uniform, deep etching pattern; however, Fuks et al. [31] found irregular etch pattern with scattered smooth areas after grinding with fine-grain silicon carbide. The latter finding may imply unequal grinding or incomplete prismless enamel removal.

In fact, clinicians face a problem in removing prismless enamel because it is clinically impossible to define its thickness. In this respect, cleaning with a rotating brush with or without fine-grain pastes is usually recommended for enamel cleaning prior to the etching procedure. This procedure provides cleaning in combination with enamel safety. Milling of the outermost enamel by various media should be avoided.

Enamel Conditioning

Phosphoric Acid

Etching of enamel with water solutions of phosphoric acid prior to the placement of resinous materials remains the most commonly used enamel conditioning. Various features, characteristics of the deciduous but not of the permanent enamel, account for considerable differences in etching efficiency and bonding capacity between deciduous and permanent teeth.

In primary teeth, the prismless layer of the enamel, which covers the buccal and lingual surfaces, the smaller enamel thickness, the higher porosity and the hypomineralization are the major characteristics of a unique enamel substrate.

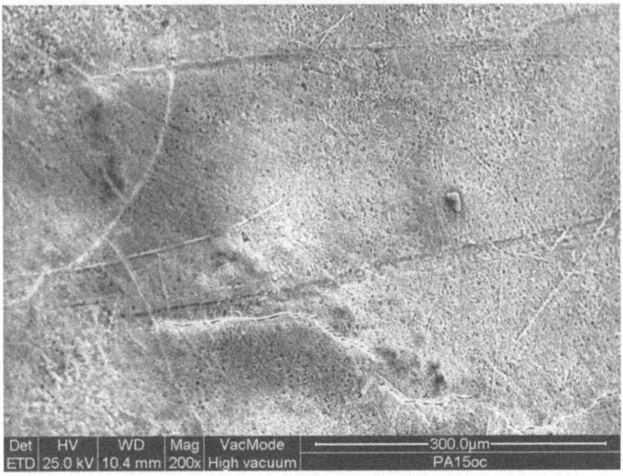

Fig. 2.1. Occlusal part of labial enamel in primary molar after etching, for 15 s, with 36 % solution of phosphoric acid. A slight porosity is obvious

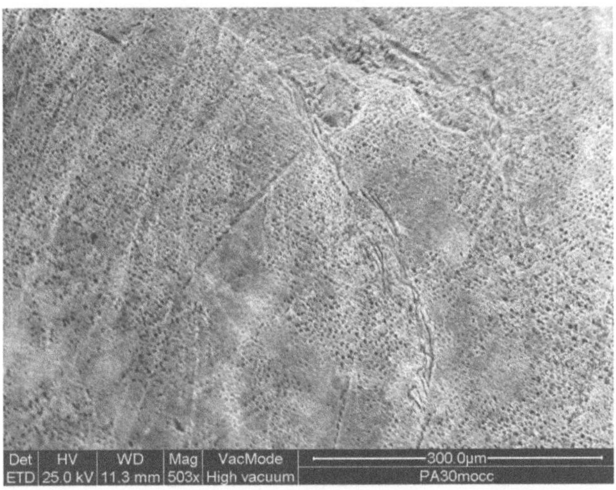

Fig. 2.2. Occlusal part of labial enamel in primary molar after etching, for 30 s, with 36 % solution of phosphoric acid. Smooth islands (acid resistant) are visible on the porous surface (acid-dissolved)

The etching patterns obtained by phosphoric acid conditioning, the optimum etching time and the bond resistance of the resinous materials have recently attracted interest and research.

Generally, the prismless outer layer is believed to reduce the effectiveness of acid etching. The higher density of the crystals and the uni-directional orientation in prismless enamel may reduce the enamel solubility, resulting in relatively unaffected enamel. If dissolution occurs, no rod patterns are displayed by preferential loss [9]; thus, enamel porosity generated by etching may not be sufficient to achieve a considerable number of resinous tags (Fig. 2.1).

Several types of acid-resistant prismless enamel, such as easily acid-dissolved and strong acid-resistant types, comprise the primary enamel (Fig. 2.2). Moreover, one dominant primary enamel etching pattern cannot be predicted since core and

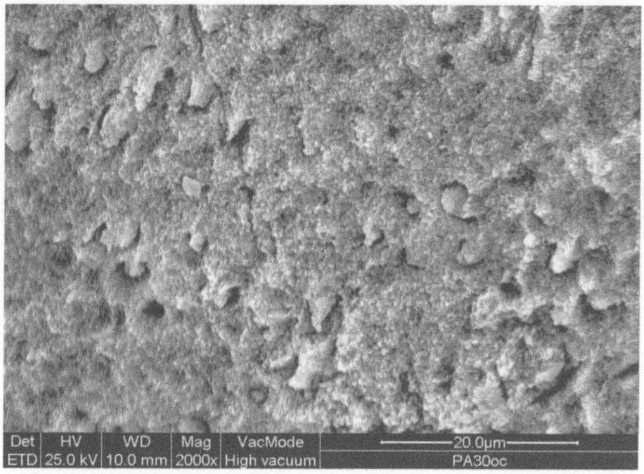
Det HV WD Mag VacMode
ETD 25.0 kV 10.0 mm 2000x High vacuum
20.0µm
PA30oc

Fig. 2.3. Occlusal part of labial enamel in primary molar after etching, for 15 s, with a 36% solution of phosphoric acid. Various etching patterns are noted

peripheral types of dissolution are equally probable [32]; therefore, conflict data have been presented concerning the etching pattern yielded on deciduous enamel. Although type-III etching, as described by Silverstone et al. [59], is considered the predominant pattern, types II and I have been frequently observed as well (Fig. 2.3) [33]. The etching pattern depends on the crystalline orientation within the single prism. Type-III pattern has often been predominant in regions where the rods are more disoriented, such as in the primary enamel. The clinical significance of each of the three etching patterns is not known, because the clinician cannot verify the pattern by visual examination and therefore cannot correlate it with the clinical success rate.

Poorly structured etching patterns, rather than peripheral ones, have been identified on unground enamel after 30- and 60-s phosphoric acid etching [26]. Controversial aspects have been drawn regarding the etching generated on ground enamel [18, 34]. The peripheral etching pattern, as a result of loss of intraprismatic structure, is the most common pattern for outer- and inner-ground primary enamel, in various tooth locations. It can be assumed that unground enamel is less resistant to acid effect. Parts of the same tooth seem to influence the etching quality as well (Fig. 2.4). Nevertheless, even in less readily etched enamel, a crystal-level etched pattern can be obtained [35]; therefore, the microfine irregularity resulting from the individual enamel crystals may provide comparable bond strength with the preferential loss of prism periphery substrate [36].

Besides, the relationship between the type of etching (well-developed, clear prism structure after etching or crystals with mild or slight etching) and the resin adhesion remains unclear [36–39]. Generally, the length of the resin tags has been shown to contribute little to the bond strength [40, 41].

Etching time is considered a major variable for the etching procedure. A wide range – 15 s to 4 min – of optimum etching times for primary enamel has been advocated [42–44]. In the early 1970s, long etching times up to 120 s were suggested as an attempt to remove the prismless enamel; however, the longer the etching time, the greater is the possibility for over-etching and for salivary contamination, particularly in young children [16, 43, 45]. In addition, it has been shown that the

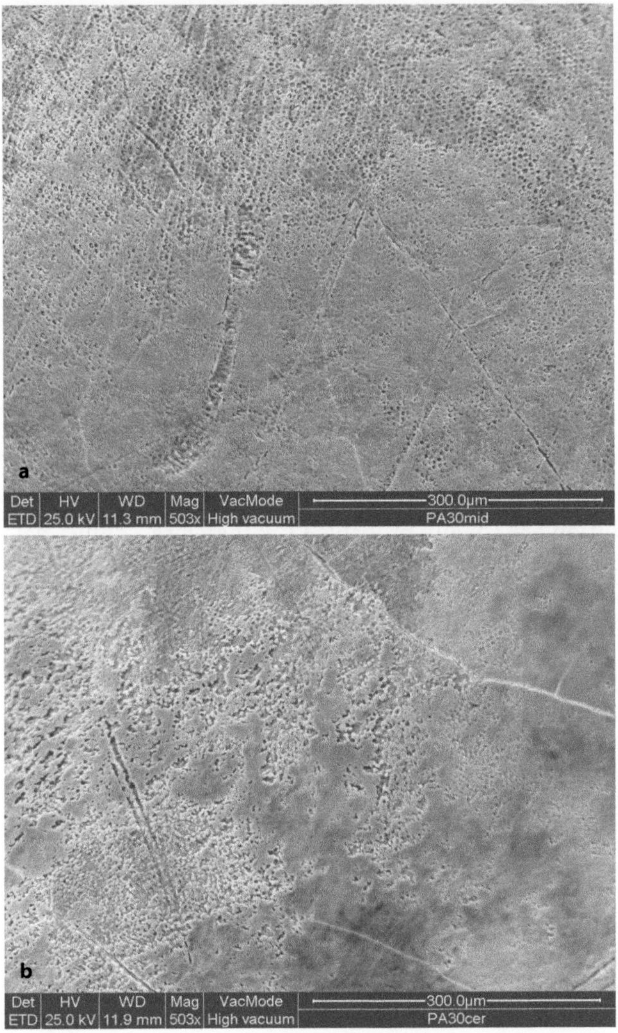

Fig. 2.4. Middle (**a**) and cervical (**b**) parts from a labial enamel in primary molar after etching, for 30 s, with 36 % solution of phosphoric acid. Differences in etching pattern can be easily verified

shorter etching time increases the rate of cases presenting etched enamel prisms [26].

Different application times of 36 % phosphoric acid induce a variety of etching patterns due to potential for heterogeneous dissolution [16]. Type-II pattern was detected after 15-s etching, whereas prism peripheries were demineralized in a homogeneous pattern after 5-s etching [46]. A tendency of type-III pattern to predominate after 15-s etching has been recorded as well [16]. At the same time, random distribution of type-I, type-II and type-III patterns were noticed [16, 47–49]. Negligible morphological changes on the enamel surface were revealed when the etching time was increased to over 30 s [33, 47]. Etching times ranged from 15 to 30 s provided a detailed etch pattern either on ground or on unground primary enamel surfaces [34, 43, 46, 50, 51]; however, more clear and deeper porosity

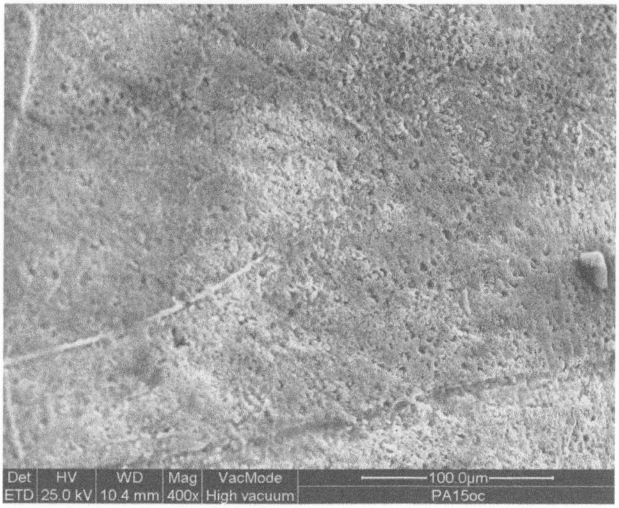

Fig. 2.5. Occlusal part of labial enamel in primary molar after etching with 36% solution of phosphoric acid, for 15 s. Comparison with Fig. 2.2 shows that shorter etching time causes milder etching effect

obtained after 30 s than after 15 s etching time (Fig. 2.5), resulting in uniform, well-performed resin projections (Fig. 2.6). Nevertheless, the retentive capacity of deciduous enamel acid conditioned for 15 s or 60 s was similar, whereas 10 s etching time caused lower bond strength [50, 52].

A completely dry enamel surface was an absolute requirement for the bonding capacity in previous generations of adhesive agents. The total-etch systems used presently require wet substrates since hydrophilic monomers function as primers and adhesives [53, 54]; therefore, the dry enamel may negatively affect the bonding efficiency.

The application of a bonding agent prior to a sealant placement, as an intermediate layer, may improve the adhesion on a substrate such as the prismless etched enamel, maximizing the surface wetting ability. The use of a bonding agent has also been suggested for a saliva-contaminated etched enamel surface, which is a common phenomenon particularly for deciduous teeth. It is well known that salivary contamination of the etched enamel surfaces results in occlusion of etching micropores (Fig. 2.7) and leads to high microleakage and low bond strength [55–57]. Saliva contamination during etching procedure induces poor sealant retention. Removal of the saliva by water rinsing and re-etching was not proved as efficient (Fig. 2.8), because of the difficulties in protein removal [58–61]. Because the currently used bonding agents are hydrophilic and were developed to bond resins to wet, hard dental tissues, it should be hypothesized that these agents may allow bonding to wet saliva-contaminated enamel surfaces as well. Increased bond strength and decrease in microleakage level were achieved when certain bonding agents from previous generation were used on both saliva-contaminated and non-contaminated surfaces [30, 55, 62]. Since the short- and long-term clinical performance of these cases has not been investigated, this cannot be suggested as a technique to deal with inadequate clinical isolation which, in fact, leads to salivary contamination.

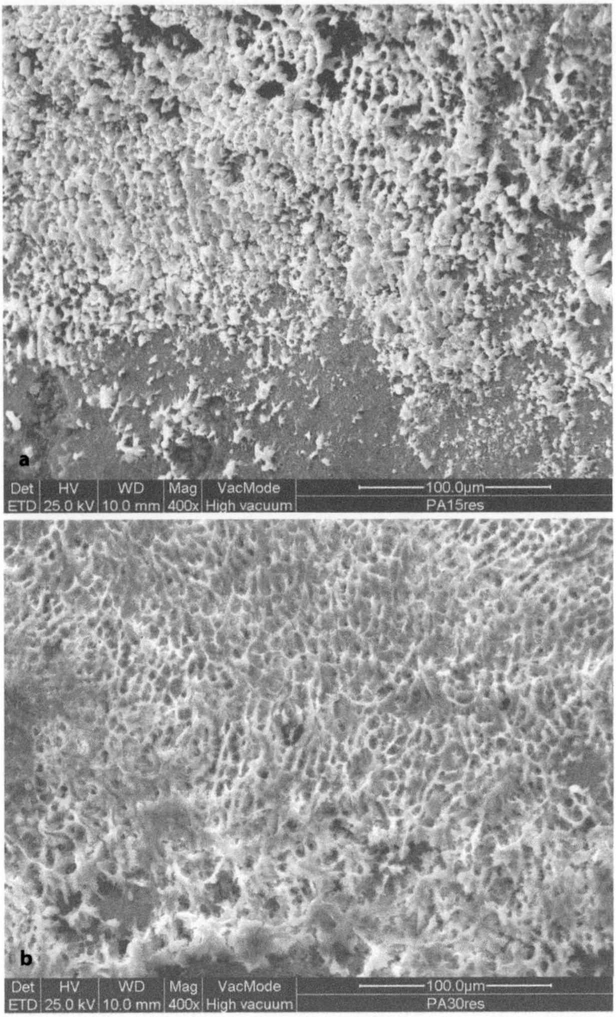

Fig. 2.6. Resin interface exposed after primary enamel dissolution (HCl 6 N, 2 h) in cases of 15 s (**a**) and 30 s (**b**) enamel etching times (36% solution of phosphoric acid). A well-performed resin network was provided by the longer etching time

Two types of phosphoric acid agents are available. The acid solutions that were first introduced have been almost completely superseded by gel analogues over the past several years. The thixotropic nature of the gels permits increased control over placement and elimination of the acid overflow.

Inferior quality of etching by acid gels compared with solutions was found (Fig. 2.9) in combination with fewer resin tags and less even distribution across the resin interface were created [63]. The viscosity of the gels may inhibit the uniform wetting ability of the agent on the enamel [64, 65]. Nevertheless, the difference in etching pattern between gel and solution acids does not reflect the resin-bonding resistance [63]. That finding may highlight the lack of correlation, under in vitro conditions, between etching quality and bond strength which can be due to different substrates used to determine the etching and the bonding efficiency.

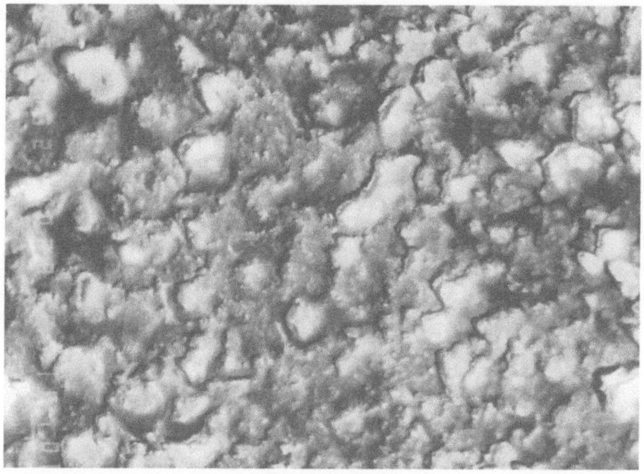

Fig. 2.7. Saliva covers the microporosity of an etched (36% solution of phosphoric acid, 30 s) primary enamel

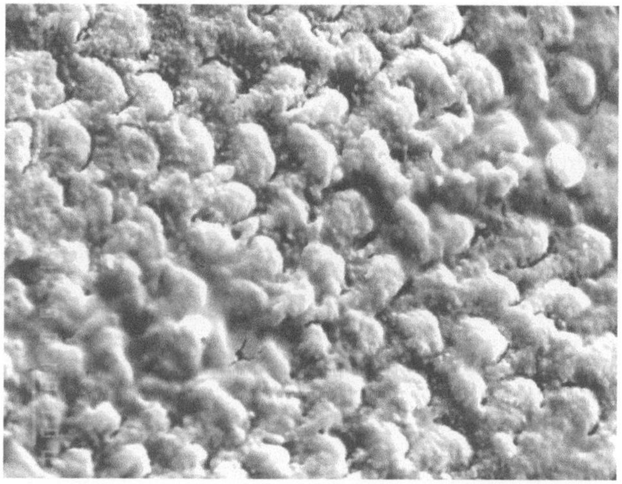

Fig. 2.8. Re-etching (15 s) of the surface shown in Fig. 2.7 recovered partially the initial etching pattern

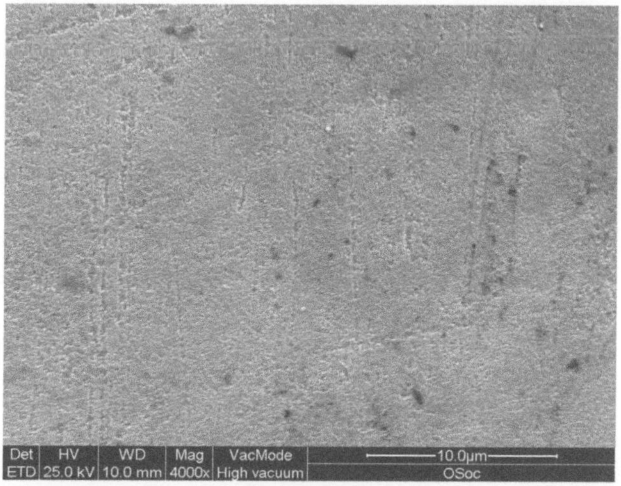

Fig. 2.9. Occlusal part of labial enamel in primary molar after etching, for 15 s, with 36% gel of phosphoric acid. A slightly pitted surface is presented

Grinding of the enamel specimens is necessary to achieve the flat surface for bonding, which results in complete prismless enamel removal. This subsurface ground enamel may be more susceptible to acid etching than the superficial prismless enamel.

Self-Etching Agents

The self-etching primers were developed to simplify the bonding procedure. These agents are based on the use of non-rinsed acidic polymerizable monomers, which serve as conditioner, primer and resin; thus, the step of enamel phosphoric acid conditioning is skipped. The use of an enamel conditioner that does not require rinsing may be a valuable clinical procedure, since satisfactory isolation may not always be possible in children. Furthermore, the self-etching priming materials can solve the problem of the relatively long time required for the various steps of the complicated adhesive procedure.

Most of the vitro studies have found that the self-etching agents provide lower bond strength to the primary enamel than the conventional enamel conditioning with phosphoric acid [66, 67]. Nevertheless, Agostini et al. [66] have reported that the bond resistance obtained is above the minimal required for permanent teeth (18.6–19.4 MPa) [68]. The short resin tags formed may cause the inferior bond strength measured [67]. It is believed that the bonding on enamel is achieved primarily not by the resinous projections but by micromechanical adhesion provided from monomer diffusion and polymerization into the microirregularities of the etched enamel (Fig. 2.10) and by formation of a hybrid-like layer [40, 41, 69]. It has been also proved, in permanent enamel, that the depth of etching, and subsequently the depth of the resin penetration induced by self-etching adhesives, is not correlated with the bond strengths attained [70, 71]; thus, the surface irregularity of the treated enamel may not be a valid indicator for the bond magnitude achieved.

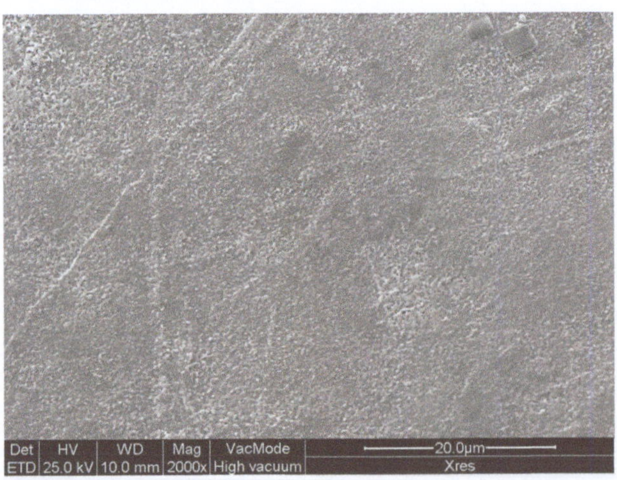

Fig. 2.10. Resin interface exposed after primary enamel dissolution (HCl 6 N, 2 h). The enamel was treated with a self-etching primer adhesive (Xeno III, Dentsply/DeTrey). Dense but short resin projections are observed

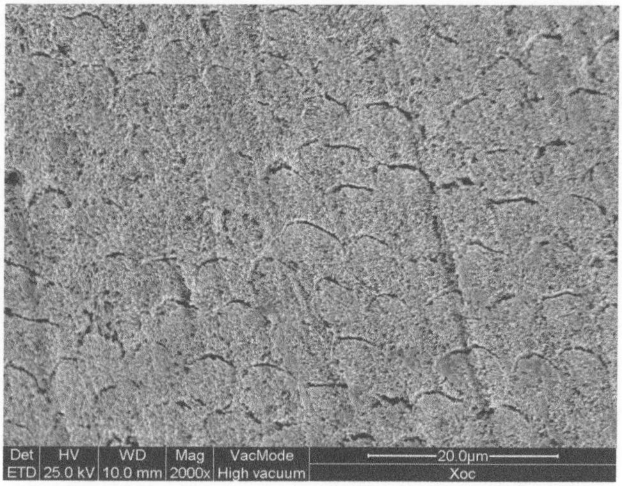

Fig. 2.11. Occlusal part of labial enamel in primary molar after treatment with a self-etching primer adhesive (Xeno III, Dentsply/DeTrey). Microirregularities have been formed on the surface

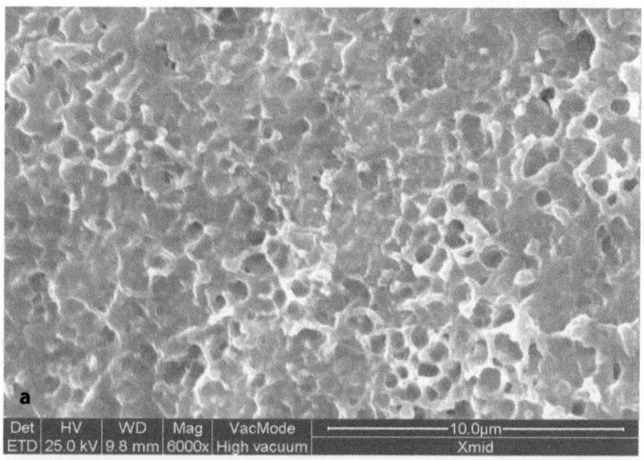

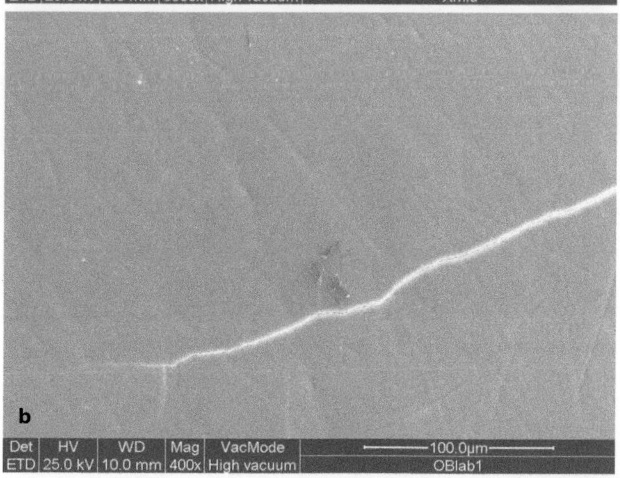

Fig. 2.12. Primary enamel treated with two different self-etching primer adhesives [Xeno III-(**a**), Dentsply/DeTrey and One Bond F-(**b**), Tokuyama]. Dissimilar etching patterns were obtained

In fact, a milder etching effect by the self-etching agents (Fig. 2.11) and a thinner bonded interface have been demonstrated than found with enamel conditioned with common phosphoric acid [67, 72]. Despite these features, no significant bond differences between the phosphoric acid and self-etching agents treated enamel surfaces has been recorded [72, 73].

The ability of the resin to penetrate into the separated superficial crystallites, which should be enveloped by the resin, may be mostly contributed to the bonding efficiency obtained. The cumulative cross-sectional interfacial area created may offer an adequate adhesive surface [74]; however, it is questionable if the shallow hybridized resin–enamel interface formed with absence of long resin tags can withstand the thermomechanical fatigue in the oral environment.

The limited number of studies concerning the use of self-etching adhesives on primary enamel and the different results generated by agents classified as self-etching (Fig. 2.12) indicate that more in vitro and clinical studies are needed to show whether or not the self-etching agents guarantee a bond to enamel.

Other Agents

In addition to the above described enamel conditioners, a few other agents have been used on primary enamel.

Citric acid (50 %) needs 5 min exposure time to give a satisfied etching pattern. This length of time is impractical, especially in children [2]. A non-rinse conditioner with main components carboxylic, maleic and itaconic acids (NRC, Dentsply/DeTrey) caused almost clear prism structure (Fig. 2.13); however, whether or not that pattern guarantees a strong and durable bond has not been adequately investigated either in vitro or in vivo [75]. The application of 10 % maleic acid for 15 s on primary enamel providing a conservative mineral loss resulted in a bond strength similar to that of permanent enamel treated with the same agent [76].

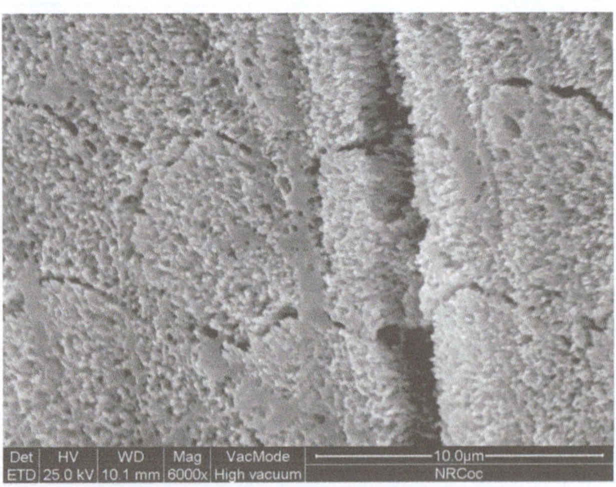

Fig. 2.13. Occlusal part of labial enamel in primary molar treated with a non-rinse conditioner (NRC, Dentsply/DeTrey)

Clinical Results

Bonding of the resinous sealants to the etched enamel facilitates the sealant retention; however, it is important to highlight that a variety of factors contribute clinically to the sealant failures. Possible reasons for sealant failures include tooth type, fissure location, sealant viscosity and wear, enamel etching efficiency, appropriate placement procedure, and regular sealant maintenance [77]; therefore, the annual rate of sealant loss reported does not reflect only the bonding effectiveness of the sealant to the etched enamel [78].

Clinical evidence suggests that sealant loss occurs in two phases. An initial early loss due to operator technique is followed by a second loss associated mostly with material wear under the forces of occlusion. The early failure frequency is considered a stronger indicator for the bonding situation obtained. Sealant loss rate within the first 2–3 months after insertion has not been assessed in clinical studies. Futatsuki et al. [79] reported a 14.4% failure rate at 2-month recall. The maxillary lingual and mandibular buccal surfaces on molars showed a higher rate of complete loss. The thicker prismless enamel found in these regions may account for this finding. Immediate bond failure between sealant and enamel is mostly attributed to saliva contamination of the enamel during and/or after enamel-etching procedure [59, 80–82]. The low ability of phosphoric acid etchant to penetrate the total fissure depth, independently of the acid viscosity, has been cited as a causative factor as well [83]. Surfactant components have been included into etchants to increase and enhance the penetration, but no research results on their efficiency are available.

Some organic remnants detected into the deep area of fissures after pumice cleaning may disturb the etchant penetration and efficiency [79]. Prolonged etching time with phosphoric acid, up to 20 s, causes no significant differences in the occlusal sealant retention in primary molars [84].

Examination of pit and fissure regions after early sealant loss revealed unetched areas along and around the observed locations as well as a mixed picture with well-etched and completely unetched spots [79].

As mentioned previously, the salivary contamination of the etched enamel surfaces negatively affects the bonding capacity of that substrate. The ability of an intermediate adhesive agent to facilitate sealant retention on etched surfaces contaminated by saliva has been shown in only one clinical study [58]. Nevertheless, the nature of the appropriate adhesive agent and the bonding mechanism induced for this antimoisture effect should be clarified for the acceptance of the suggested procedure. Despite this, the findings of that study must be interpreted with caution because of the small sample number (20 patients) examined.

An indication that the primary enamel consists of a different bonding substrate than with the permanent one is given by the early sealant failures recorded in deciduous and in permanent teeth. Due to the fact that the number of studies is limited, it cannot be inferred that there are differences in the retention rate of sealants between primary and permanent teeth [84].

References

1. Wilson P, Beynon L. Mineralization differences between human deciduous and permanent enamel measured by quantitative microradiography. J Clin Pediatr Dent 1991; 15:188–194
2. Shama A, Chanda S, Jaiswel J, Bajpai V. Effect of conditioning the enamel surface of primary teeth with citric acid: a SEM study. J Clin Pediatr Dent 1992; 16:207-212
3. Cutress T. The inorganic composition and solubility of dental enamel from several specified population groups. Arch Oral Biol 1972; 17: 93–109
4. Naujorks R, Schade H, Zelinka I. Chemical composition of different areas of the enamel of deciduous and permanent teeth (the content of Ca, P, CO_2, Na and N_2). Caries Res 1967; 1:137–143
5. Besic F, Bayard M, Wiemann M, Burrell K. Composition and structure of dental enamel: elemental composition and crystalline structure of dental enamel as they relate to its solubility. Am J Dent 1975; 91:594–601
6. Arends J, Jongebloed W. Dislocations and dissolution in apatites: theoretical considerations. Caries Res 1977; 11:186–188
7. Weatherell J, Weidman S, Nyman S. Density patterns in enamel. Caries Res 1967; 1:42–51
8. Fidelman E. The structure of the enamel in primary teeth: practical applications in restorative techniques. J Dent Child 1976; 43:172–176
9. Gwinnett A. Human prismless enamel and its influence on sealant penetration. Arch Oral Biol 1973; 18:441–444
10. Hørsted M, Fejerskov O, Larsen M, Thylstrup A. The structure of surface with special reference to occlusal surfaces in primary and permanent teeth. Caries Res 1976; 10:287–296
11. Gwinnett A. Structure and composition of enamel. Oper Dent 1992; Suppl 5:10–17
12. Gwinnett A. The ultrastructure of the "prismless" enamel of deciduous teeth. Arch Oral Biol 1966; 11:1109–1116
13. Whittaker D. Structural variations in the surface zone of human tooth enamel observed by scanning electron microscopy. Arch Oral Biol 1982; 27:383–392
14. Ripa L, Gwinnett A, Buonocore M. The "prismless" outer layer of deciduous and permanent enamel. Arch Oral Biol 1966; 11:41–48
15. Costa L, Watanale I, Fawa N. Scanning electron microscopy of prismless enamel in non-erupted deciduous teeth. Ann Braz Soc Dent Res 1994; 10:126–134
16. Costa L, Watanabe L, Fawa M. Three-Dimensional aspects of etched enamel in non-erupted deciduous teeth. Braz Dent J 1998; 9:95–100
17. Horsted M, Fejerskov O, Larsen MJ, Thylstrup A. The structure of surface enamel with special reference to occlusal surfaces of primary and permanent teeth. Caries Res 1976; 10:287–296
18. Meola M, Papaccio G. A scanning electron microscope study of the effect of etching time and mechanical pre-treatment on the pattern of acid etching on the enamel of primary teeth. Int Dent J 1986; 36:49–53
19. Lyon D, Darling A. Orientation of the crystallites in human dental enamel (I). Br Dent J 1957; 102:483–488
20. Meckel A. The formation and properties of organic films on teeth. Arch Oral Biol 1965; 10:585–597
21. Clasen A, Hanning M, Skjorland K, Sonju T. Analytical and ultrastructural studies of pellicle on primary teeth. Acta Odont Scand 1997; 55:339–343
22. Ishizaki A. Further studies and the direct bonding system. Part I: Scanning electron microscopic studies of the bonding mechanism and the effect on the tooth surface. Jpn J Orthod 1975; 32:227–237
23. Kaneko H, Imau Y, Miyazawva H, Imamishi T, Akahane S. A study on pit and fissure sealant. Jpn J Pedodont 1986; 24:1–12
24. Kuroiwa M, Nakajima F, Kodaka T. Acid-etched effects after some preparations of enamel surfaces in human deciduous teeth. J Showa Univ Dent Soc 1984; 3:221–226

25. Hosoya Y, Johnston J. Evaluation of various cleaning and polishing methods on primary enamel. J Periodont 1989; 13:253–269
26. Hosoya Y, Goto G. The effects of cleaning, polishing pretreaments and acid etching times on unground primary enamel. J Periodont 1990; 14:84–92
27. Waggoner W, Slegal M. Pit and fissure. Sealant application: updating the technique. J Am Dent Assoc 1996; 127:351–361
28. Main C, Thomson J, Cummings A, Field D, Stephen K, Gillespie F. Surface treatment studies aimed at streamlining fissure sealant application. J Oral Rehabil 1983; 10:307–317
29. Schuermer E, Burgess J, Matis B. Strength of bond of composite resin to enamel cleaned with a paste containing fluoride. Gen Dent 1990; 38:381–383
30. Fritz V, Garcia-Godoy F, Finger W. Enamel and dentin bond strength and bonding mechanism to dentin of Gluma CPS to primary teeth. J Dent Child 1997; 64:32–38
31. Fuks A, Eidelman E, Shapira J. Mechanical and acid treatment of the prismless layer of primary teeth vs acid etching only: a SEM study. ASDC J Dent Child 1977; 44:222–225
32. Bozalis W, Marshall W. Acid etching patterns of primary enamel. J Dent Res 1977; 56:185
33. Hosoya Y. The effect of acid etching times on ground primary enamel. J Clin Pediatr Dent 1991; 15:188–194
34. Simonsen R. Fissure sealants: deciduous molar retention of colored sealant with variable etch time. Quintessence Int 1978; 9:71–77
35. Tyler J. A scanning electron microscope study of factors influencing etch patterns of human enamel. Arch Oral Biol 1976; 21:765–769
36. Tegami J. Effects of acid etching technique of adhesion of the composite resin applied to the enamel. Kobyooshi 1983; 50:533–567
37. Luse K. Studies on bond strength of composite resin to the acid-etched enamel. Jpn J Conserve Dent 1978; 29:326–349
38. Ogawa J. Scanning electron microscopic study of enamel treatment and resin bonding strength. Jpn J Conserv Dent 1986; 29:813–842
39. Xu Hc, Wang T, Wang H. A study of the state and depth of resin penetration into acid-etched enamel. Austral Dent J 1983; 28:359–365
40. Kanemura N, Sano H, Tagami J. Tensile bond strength to and SEM evaluation of ground and intact enamel surfaces. J Dent 1999; 27:523–530
41. Shinchi M, Soma K, Nakabayashi N. The effect of phosphoric acid concentration on resin tag length and bond strength of a photo-cured resin to acid etched enamel. Dent Mater 2000;16:324–329
42. Bozalis W, Marshall G, Cooley R. Mechanical pretreatments and etching of primary tooth enamel. J Dent Child 1979; 43:43–49
43. Hosoya Y. Resin adhesion to the ground young permanent enamel: surface of etching times and thermal cycling test. J Clin Pediatr Dent 1994; 18:115–121
44. Myers D, Butts M. Surface topography of the cavosurface enamel bevel following and etching in primary teeth. J Pedodont 1985; 10:63–67
45. Redford D, Clarkson B, Jensen M. The effect of different etching times on the sealant bond strength, etch depth and pattern in primary teeth. Pediatr Dent 1986; 8:11–15
46. Tandon S, Kumari R, Udupa S. The effect of etch-time on the bond strength of a sealant and on the etch pattern in primary and permanent enamel: an evaluation. J Dent Child 1989; 3:186–190
47. Garcia-Godoy F, Gwinnett A. Effect of etching times and mechanical pretreatment on the enamel of primary teeth: an SEM study. Am J Dent 1991; 4:115–118
48. Nordenvall KJ, Brännström M, Malmgren O. Etching of deciduous teeth and young and old teeth. A comparison between 15 and 60 seconds of etching. Am J Orthod 1980; 78:99–108
49. Tinanoff N, Mueller B. Acid etch characteristics on prismless enamel. J Int Assoc Dent Child 1997; 8:17–21
50. Hosoya V, Goto G. Resin adhesion to the ground primary enamel: influence of etching times and thermal cycling test. J Clin Pediatr Dent 1992; 17:25–31
51. Nyers D, Butts M. Surface topography of the cavosurface enamel level following acid etching in primary teeth. J Periodont 1985; 10:63–67

52. Gwinnett A, Garcia-Godoy F. Effect of etching time and acid concentration on resin shear bond strength to primary tooth enamel. Am J Dent 1992; 5:237–239
53. Hosoya Y, Nakanura N, Shmagawa H, Goto G. Resin adhesion to the ground enamel: influence of the ground depths of the enamel and etching times (I). Jpn J Pedodont 1989; 27:922–935
54. Sun C. Relationship between length of resin tag and bond strength of bonding adhesive. J Fuianoka Dent Coll 1990; 17:383–399
55. Bomem L, Feigal R. Reducing microleakage of sealants under salivary contamination digital-image analysis evaluation. Quintessence Int 1994; 25:283
56. Borem L, Feigal R. Reducing microleakage of sealants under salivary contamination: digital-image analysis evaluation. Quintessence Int 1994; 25:283–289
57. Mitt J, Feigal R. Use of a bonding agent to reduce sealant sensitivity to moisture contamination: an in vitro study. Pediatr Dent 1992; 14:41–46
58. Feigal R, Hitt J, Splieth C. Retaining sealant on salivary contamination enamel. J Am Dent Assoc 1993; 124:88–96
59. Silverstone L, Hicks M, Featherstone M. Oral fluid contamination of etched enamel surfaces. A SEM study. J Am Dent Assoc 1985; 110:329–332
60. Thomson JL, Main C, Gillespie FC, Stephen KW. The effects of salivary contamination on fissure sealant-enamel bond strength. J Oral Rehabil 1981; 8:11–18
61. Xie J, Powers J, McGuekin R. In vitro bond strength of two adhesives to enamel and dentin under normal and contaminated conditions. Dent Mater 1993; 9:295–299
62. Grande R, Ballester R, Singer J, Santos J. Microleakage of a universal adhesive used as a fissure sealant. Am J Dent 1998; 11:109–113
63. Walker M, Vann W. In vitro comparison of primary incisor enamel surfaces etched with an acid solution or acid gel. Pediatr Dent 1984; 6:209–213
64. Gwinnett A. Acid etching for composite resin. Dent Clin North Am 1981; 25:271–289
65. Moin K, Dogan I. Indirect bonding of orthodontic attachments. Am J Orthod 1977; 72:161–175
66. Agostini F, Kaaden C, Powers J. Bond strength of self-etching primers to enamel and dentin of primary teeth. Pediatr Dent 2001; 23:481–486
67. Hosoya Y, Kawashita Y, Yoshiba M, Suefuji C, Marshall G. Fluoridated light-activated bonding resin adhesion to enamel and dentin: primary vs. permanent. Pediatr Dent 2000; 22:101–106
68. Retief D, Mandras R, Russell C. Shear bond strength required to prevent microleakage at the dentin–resin interface. Am J Dent 1994; 7:43–46
69. Nakabayashi N, Kojima K, Masuhara E. The promotion of adhesion by the infiltration of monomers into tooth substrates. J Biomed Mater Res 1982; 16:265–273
70. Barkmeter W, Los A, Triolo P. Bond strength and SEM evaluation of Clearfil Liner Bond 2. Am J Dent 1995; 8:289–293
71. Pedrigâo J, Lopes L, Lambrechis P, Leitâo J, Van Meerbeck B, Vanherle G. Effect of self-etching primer on enamel shear bond strengths and SEM morphology. Am J Dent 1977; 10:141–146
72. Shimada Y, Senawongse P, Harnirattisai C, Burrow M, Nakaoki Y, Tagami J. Bond strength of two adhesive systems to primary and permanent enamel. Oper Dent 2002; 27:403–409
73. Hosoya Y, Tominaga A. A comparison of five adhesive systems to primary enamel. Pediatr Dent 1999; 21:46–52
74. Nakabayashi N, Pashley D (eds) Acid conditioning and hybridization of substrates. In: Hybridization of dental hard tissues. Quintessence, Tokyo, 1998; pp 37–56
75. Cehreli Z, Altay N. Etching effect of 17% EDTA and a non-rinse conditioner (NRC) on primary enamel and dentin. Am J Dent 2000; 13:64–68
76. Hallett K, Garcia-Godoy F, Trotter A. Shear bond strength of a resin composite to enamel etched with maleic of phosphoric acid. Austr Dent J 1994; 39:292–297
77. Simonsen R. Pit and fissure sealant: review of the literature. Pediatr Dent 2002; 24:393–414
78. Feigal R. Sealants and preventive restorations: review of effectiveness and clinical changes for improvement. Pediatr Dent 1998; 20:85–92
79. Futatsuki M, Kubota K, Yeh Y, Park K, Moss S. Early loss of pit and fissure sealant: a clinical and SEM study. J Clin Pediatr Dent 1995; 19:99–104

80. Hormati A, Fuller J, Denehy G. Effects of contamination and mechanical disturbance on the quality of acid-etched enamel. J Am Dent Assoc 1980; 100:34–38
81. Gwinnett A. Bonding of restorative resins to enamel. Ind Dent J 1988; 38:91–95
82. Simonsen R. The clinical effectiveness of a colored pit and fissure sealant at 36 months. J Am Dent Assoc 1981; 102:323–327
83. Bottenberg P, Graber HG, Lampert I. Penetration of etching agents and its influence on sealer penetration into fissures in vitro. Dent Mater 1996; 12:96–102
84. Simonsen R. Fissure sealants in primary molars: retention of colored sealants with variable etch times, at 12 months. J Dent Child 1979; 46:382–384

Bond Strength to Enamel

3

J. M. Powers, W.H. Tate

Introduction

The ability of the clinician to bond restorative materials to enamel has been an important achievement of modern dentistry. A variety of restorative materials that rely on enamel bonding are now available to the clinician. These materials include resin composites, compomers, hybrid ionomers, and glass ionomers.

In this chapter, in vitro bond testing is discussed as well as the effects of variables that affect bond strength to enamel. From a clinical perspective, retention rates of materials bonded to enamel is discussed, with examples from studies of porcelain veneers, pit-and-fissure sealants and orthodontic bonding.

Measurement of Bond Strength

In vitro measurements of debonding force and bond strength are important in characterizing the bonding potential of new adhesives and restorative materials to enamel. The first goal of bond testing is to measure the force of debonding relative to a bonded area. The second goal is to observe the location of the bond failure.

Debonding Force

The debonding force is measured in units of newtons (N), kilograms (kg), or pounds (lb). This force must then be related to the nominal area of bonding. Typically, diameters of bonded specimens reported in the research literature vary from 1 to 4.5 mm, representing bonded areas of 0.8–15.9 mm^2. In general, specimens tested with smaller bonded areas result in higher values of bond strength.

Bond Strength

Bond strength, which is the force of debonding divided by the nominal area of the bonded interface, is commonly reported in the literature in units of megapascals (MPa), kilograms per square centimeter (kg/cm^2), and pounds per square inch (lb/in^2 or psi).

Table 3.1. Hypothetical in vitro tensile bond strengths of resin composite bonded to enamel

Resin Composite	Bond strength (MPa)	Failure location (%)
A	8	100 – adhesive
B	18	100 – cohesive in resin composite
C	26	100 – cohesive in enamel

Bond Failure

Adhesive failures are those that occur between the adhesive and the tooth. Cohesive failures can occur within the tooth or within the restorative material. Bond failures are often a mixture of adhesive and cohesive failures. The percentages of the types of bond failure can be measured using a scale that specifies the amount (in percent) of restorative material remaining on the tooth after debonding.

For example, a hypothetical bond strength experiment (Table 3.1) found that resin composite A had 100% adhesive failures at the enamel/resin composite interface, whereas resin composite B had 100% cohesive failures in the resin composite and resin composite C had 100% cohesive failures in the enamel substrate.

In this experiment, the bond strength of resin composite A was lower than its cohesive strength and the resin composite separated cleanly from the tooth. The relatively low bond strength of resin composite A might suggest that this resin composite bonds poorly to enamel, or that the enamel surface was contaminated, resulting in an inferior bond. In contrast, there were cohesive failures in the resin composite for resin composite B and in the enamel substrate for resin composite C. The relatively high values of "bond strength" demonstrate that these resin composites bonded well to enamel, although the actual values of bond strength are not known; however, the 100% cohesive failure in resin composite B might indicate that it was poorly polymerized. The 100% cohesive failure in the enamel substrate for resin composite C might indicate that the enamel substrate was thin or cracked.

Bond Strength Measurement by Tensile and Shear Testing

Bond strength testing typically is performed in tension or shear, using a screw-driven or servohydraulic universal testing machine [1]. In tensile testing the restorative material is pulled perpendicularly from the enamel substrate. Two popular tensile bond tests include the inverted, truncated cone test (Fig. 3.1) [2] and the microtensile test (Fig. 3.2) [3]. In a study of two bonding agents bonded to enamel, superficial dentin and deep dentin for wet, moist, and dry conditions, microtensile bond strengths were found overall to be approximately 30% higher than inverted cone bond strengths (p=0.002, r^2=0.45; Table 3.2) [4]. The higher bond strengths observed with the microtensile test may be related to the smaller diameter of the bonded interface.

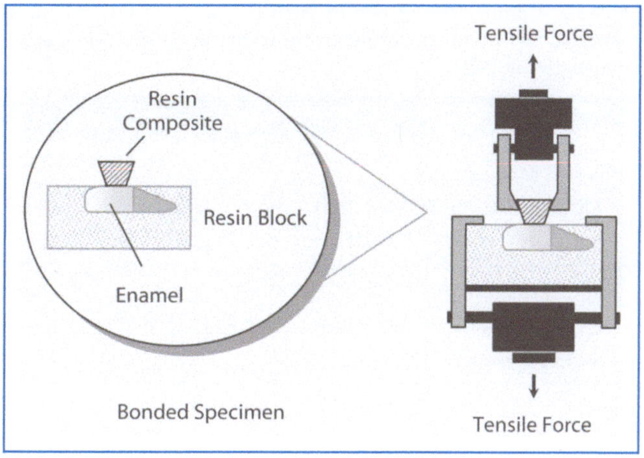

Fig. 3.1. Test assembly (isolated interface model) for debonding adhesive from human enamel in tension. (From [15])

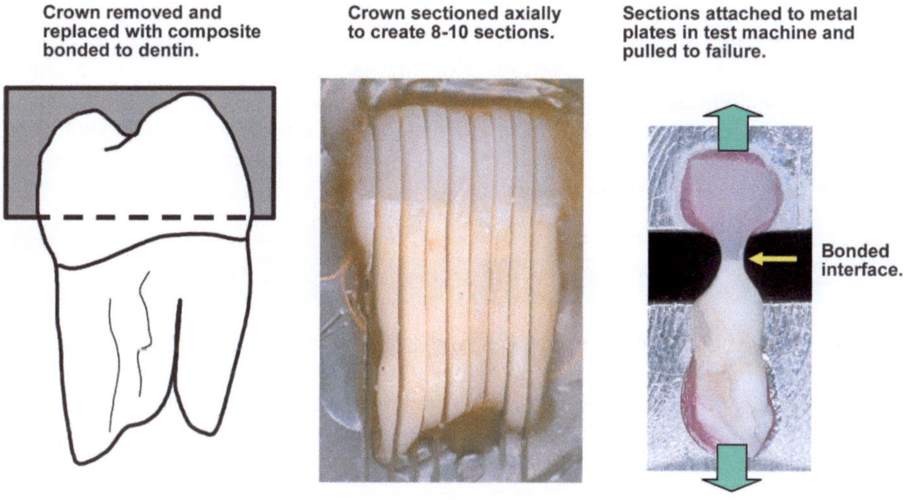

Fig. 3.2. Test assembly for microtensile bond test. (From [1])

In shear testing, the bonded bracket is loaded by a blade in tension or compression or by a wire loop in tension, so that the bracket slides parallel to the enamel surface [1]. Pure shear loading is difficult to achieve, and most shear testing also includes components of peeling, tension, and torsion.

Both tensile and shear loading modes are valid tests for studying bond strengths of restorative materials. The goal in bond testing should be to achieve a coefficient of variation [(standard deviation/mean) × 100%] in the range of 20–30%. Typically, tensile testing produces a lower coefficient of variation than the most common shear tests.

Table 3.2. Comparison of two in vitro tensile bond tests for measurement of bond strengths (MPa) of two bonding agents and a resin composite bonded to wet, moist, and dry human enamel. (From [4])

Bonding agent	Wet	Moist	Dry
Inverted cone tensile test			
Fifth generation (Single Bond)	21.0	20.2	26.6
Sixth generation (EXL 542)	20.2	25.0	19.8
Microtensile test			
Fifth generation (Single Bond)	31.6	38.5	32.2
Sixth generation (EXL 542)	15.7	24.5	14.8

Bond testing using teeth involves many variables that can affect the measured bond strength. These variables include: (a) type of tooth (e.g., incisor, molar, human, bovine); (b) fluoride content of tooth; (c) disinfection and storage media of tooth before bonding; (d) elapsed time of storage following bonding; (e) type of loading (shear, tension); (f) configuration of specimen testing jig; (g) crosshead speed of mechanical testing machine; and (h) bonding area of the specimen. A technical specification (dental materials – testing of adhesion to tooth structure, ISO/TS 11405 N355) currently is under development to standardize testing protocols for bond strength measurements.

Experimental Models for Evaluating Bond Strength

Evaluation of bond strength can be studied in vitro using a simulated clinical model. A more fundamental test is the isolated substrate model in which bonding of an adhesive-to-tooth structure or a restorative material is studied independently. Retention of restorations or bond failures can be studied clinically using prospective or retrospective clinical models.

Clinical Simulation Model

In this model, for example, an orthodontic bracket would be bonded to an extracted tooth using an orthodontic resin cement [5]. Then, the bracket–tooth system would be loaded in a testing machine to cause a bond failure. This technique appears to be clinically relevant. The disadvantage of this simulated test is that bond failures often occur at several interfaces (bracket/cement, tooth/cement), so it is difficult to isolate variables that may affect bond failure.

Table 3.3. Summary of advantages and disadvantages of prospective and retrospective clinical studies. (From [6])

Type of study	Advantages	Disadvantages
Prospective	Randomization reduces bias	Patients lose choice of treatment
	Conclusions may be stronger	Patients may drop out of study
		Ethical concerns if one treatment is perceived as inferior
Retrospective	Minimal expenses	Variations in patients may cause confounding effects
	Easy to perform (record review)	Interpretation of charts (possible bias)

Isolated Interface Model

In this model, the adhesive/enamel interface is studied separately by bonding a cylinder or cone of restorative material or cement directly to the enamel surface and then debonding the restorative material or cement (Fig. 3.1) [5].

Clinical Studies

The randomized clinical trial is an experimental study in which the investigator selects and controls the treatments under study in order to draw conclusions about whether a particular treatment produced an effect [6]. The converse of the prospective study is the retrospective (observational) study, which involves the examination of previous treatment records to obtain data for analysis. The investigator thus obtains research data by observing treatment events without controlling them. Advantages and disadvantages of prospective and retrospective clinical studies are summarized in Table 3.3 [6].

Variables Affecting In Vitro Bond Strength

Differences Among Teeth

Differences in shear bond strength among maxillary teeth (6–13 MPa) and among mandibular teeth (9–13 MPa) have been reported [7]. Permanent teeth tend to produce similar or slightly higher bond strengths than primary teeth (Table 3.4) [8–10].

Table 3.4. In vitro tensile bond strengths (MPa) of self-etching adhesive systems and resin composite to human enamel

Adhesive system	Permanent[a]	Primary[b]
Self-etching primer and adhesive (Clearfil SE Bond)	29	19
Self-etching adhesive (Prompt L-Pop)	22	19

[a] From [8].
[b] From [9].

Table 3.5. Range of in vitro tensile bond strengths (MPa) of resin composite with four generations of bonding agents bonded to moist human enamel and superficial dentin. (From [14])

Bonding agent	Enamel	Superficial dentin
Fourth generation	23–32	21–24
Fifth generation	19–33	18–22
Sixth generation	17–29	17–35
Seventh generation[a]	22	15

[a] J.M. Powers and L.M. Pinzon, unpublished data.

Phosphoric Acid

In restorative dentistry the highest possible bond strength to tooth structure is desirable. Bond strengths of resin composites used with fourth-, fifth-, sixth-, and seventh-generation bonding agents to human enamel and dentin are considered satisfactory [11–14]. Generally, bond strengths to enamel are higher than those to superficial dentin (Table 3.5). Additional information on sixth- and seventh-generation bonding agents is presented in the next section of this chapter.

In contrast, the orthodontic bond strength must be sufficient to retain the brackets but low enough to allow easy cleanup of adhesive when the case is completed and the brackets are removed. Some factors that influence acid etching of enamel for orthodontic bonding include the type and concentration of the acid and the time of etching [6].

Compomers (polyacid-modified resins) bond well to enamel (Table 3.6) [15]. The highest bond strengths are achieved with the use of phosphoric acid etching and a bonding agent, although there is limited bonding of the compomer by itself to moist enamel.

Hybrid ionomers (resin-modified glass ionomers) also bond to enamel (Table 3.7) [16]. The highest bond strengths of hybrid ionomers to enamel are observed when the enamel is etched with phosphoric acid. Etching with a polyacrylic acid conditioner (10 or 20%) typically produces lower bond strengths than etching with phosphoric acid. Some hybrid ionomers are self-adhesive, although bond strengths are usually <15 MPa.

Table 3.6. In vitro tensile bond strengths (MPa) of a compomer (Compoglass F) bonded to moist and wet human enamel as affected by etching with phosphoric acid and use of a bonding agent. (From [15])

Phosphoric acid	Bonding agent*	Moist	Wet
Yes	Yes	20.3[a]	19.8[a]
Yes	No	15.5[b]	0.0
No	Yes	15.2[b]	10.8
No	No	3.5	0.0

* Syntac Single-Component; the same superscript letter means statistically the same (p=0.05).

Table 3.7. In vitro tensile bond strengths (MPa) of hybrid ionomers bonded to human enamel as affected by etching with phosphoric acid. [From (16)]

Phosphoric acid	Fuji Ortho	Fuji Ortho LC	Vitremer
Yes	26.7[a]	22.1	16.8
No	25.4[a]	14.6	8.4

[a] The same superscript letter means statistically the same (p=0.05).

Table 3.8. In vitro tensile bond strengths (MPa) of a resin composite bonded to human enamel treated with a self-etching bonding agent. [From (8)]

Resin Composite	Enamel	Superficial Dentin	Deep Dentin
Adper Prompt L-Pop	22.4	8.4	5.7
Clearfil SE Bond	29.1	27.3	20.2
Etch & Prime	21.5	3.2	1.3

Acidic Primers and Adhesives

An alternative to etching enamel with phosphoric acid is to use self-etching bonding agents, often referred to as sixth- or seventh-generation bonding agents. The sixth-generation bonding agents include the self-etching primer and adhesive (apply primer, then apply adhesive) and the self-etching adhesive (mix components, then apply adhesive). The seventh-generation bonding agents are no-mix, self-etching adhesives (apply adhesive). With these bonding agents, no phosphoric acid is used and no rinsing is necessary, and bond strengths to enamel and superficial dentin can be adequate (Table 3.8) [8].

Several fifth-generation bonding agents (One-Step Plus, Optibond Solo Plus) have the option of using either phosphoric acid or a self-etching primer before application of the adhesive. In general, the bond strengths are comparable (Table 3.9). [17].

Table 3.9. In vitro tensile bond strengths (MPa) of resin composites bonded to human enamel treated with either phosphoric acid or a self-priming etchant and a fifth-generation bonding agent. (From [17])

Resin Composite	Phosphoric acid/One-Step Plus	Tyrian SPE/One-Step Plus
Filtek Z250	19.4	19.1
TPH Spectrum	17.7	16.3
Tetric Ceram HB	18.6	17.0

Table 3.10. In vitro tensile bond strengths (MPa) of light-cured (Transbond) or self-cured (Concise Orthodontic) orthodontic resin cements bonded to human enamel treated with self-etching bonding agents. (From [18])

Bonding agent	Light-cured cement	Self-cured cement
Phosphoric acid (control)	12.9	21.4
Self-etching primer+adhesive (Clearfil SE Bond)	22.7	13.3
Self-etching adhesive (Prompt L-Pop)	17.0	0.0
Fifth-generation adhesive (Prime & Bond NT)	10.1	0.0

The bond strength of light-cured bonding agents can be affected by the use of self-cured resins. In particular, bonding agents with acidic components may exhibit reduced bond strengths with a self-cured, orthodontic resin cement (Table 3.10) [18].

Fluoride

Teeth with a higher concentration of fluoride are generally considered more resistant to acid etching than normal teeth and may require an extended etching time. In vitro bond strengths of sealants bonded to human enamel do not appear to be greatly affected by various fluoride treatments (Table 3.11) [19].

Table 3.11. In vitro tensile bond strengths (MPa) of pit-and-fissure resin sealants to human enamel treated with fluoride. (From [19])

Fluoride treatment	Unfilled sealant	Filled sealant
Control (saliva)	15^{a}	24^{c}
NaF	21^{b}	19^{d}
SnF2	14^{a}	$22^{c,d}$
APF	$18^{a,b}$	18^{d}

The same superscript letter means statistically the same (p=0.05).

Table 3.12. In vitro microtensile bond strength (MPa) of a resin composite bonded to prepared and intact enamel treated with self-etching adhesive systems. (From [21])

Adhesive system	Prepared enamel	Intact enamel
Phosphoric acid/Single Bond (control)	34.9[a]	31.5[a]
Adper Prompt L-Pop	16.6	11.8
Clearfil SE Bond	20.4[b]	16.7[b]
One-Up Bond F	10.0	0.1

The same superscript letter means statistically the same ($p=0.05$).

Table 3.13. In vitro tensile bond strength (MPa) of orthodontic resin cements to prepared and intact enamel treated with self-etching orthodontic adhesive systems

Adhesive system	Prepared enamel[a]	Intact enamel[b]
Phosphoric acid/Transbond(control)	26	35
First Step	25	20
Ideal 1	12	9
Transbond Plus	25	18

[a] From [22].
[b] From [23].

Intact Enamel

Manufacturers of sixth- and seventh-generation bonding agents (self-etching primers and self-etching adhesives) usually recommend bonding to enamel prepared (ground) with an abrasive instrument (carbide bur or diamond) or etching the intact (unground) enamel with phosphoric acid first. Research suggests that bonding to intact enamel with a self-etching bonding agent can result in a reduction in the bond strength as compared with prepared enamel (Tables 3.12, 3.13) [20–23]. Conversely, a recent study that evaluated bond strength of self-etching adhesives to bovine enamel showed no effect of prepared vs intact enamel [24]. Phosphoric acid etching produces good bonds to both prepared and intact enamel [20, 21].

Caries-Like Lesions

The highest bond strengths are achieved with sound enamel. A caries-like lesion resulted in a reduction in bond strength of 38–58% (Table 3.14) [25].

Table 3.14. In vitro tensile bond strengths (MPa) of resin composite and fourth-generation bonding agent to sound human enamel or enamel with caries-like lesion. (From [25])

Phosphoric acid	Sound enamel	Caries-like lesion
Yes	24	12
No	15	5

Table 3.15. In vitro tensile bond strengths (MPa) of a fifth-generation bonding agent and a resin composite bonded to human enamel prepared with air abrasion with or without etching with phosphoric acid. (From A.B. Matos et al., unpublished data)

Acid etched	Control	Particle size of alumina (mm)	
		27	50
Yes	23.8	23.8	15.6
No	9.5	9.3	12.0

Table 3.16. In vitro tensile bond strengths (MPa) of a hybrid ionomer bonded to human enamel prepared with air abrasion and with or without conditioning with 10% polyacrylic acid. (From [27])

Conditioned	Control	Air pressure of 27 µm, particles (psi)		
		80	120	160
Yes	14.4[a]	12.9[a]	17.9[b]	17.1[b]
No	–	2.9	10.1[c]	10.5[c]

The same superscript letter means statistically the same (p=0.05).

Air Abrasion

Air abrasion, also referred to as micro-etching, is a technique in which particles of aluminum oxide are propelled against the surface of enamel or other substrate by high air pressure, causing abrasion of the surface. Some manufacturers of commercial units have suggested that air abrasion could eliminate acid etching; however, bond strengths to air-abraded enamel are only approximately 50% of those to acid-etched enamel for resin composites (Table 3.15) [26] and hybrid ionomers (Table 3.16) [27].

Table 3.17. In vitro tensile bond strengths (MPa) of a resin composite bonded to human enamel prepared with either a carbide bur or an Erbium:YAG laser and treated with phosphoric acid/bonding agent, a self-etching adhesive, or bonding agent with no etchant. (From [29])

Etching condition	Carbide Bur	Erbium:YAG laser
Phosphoric acid/bonding agent	25.4[a]	25.8[a]
Self-etching adhesive	16.9	10.8
Bonding agent with no etchant	0.0	16.7

The same superscript letter means statistically the same (p=0.05).

Laser Etching

Bond strengths of enamel prepared with phosphoric acid etching are higher than those of enamel prepared with an Erbium-YAG laser (Table 3.17) [28, 29].

Moisture and Contaminants

Moist teeth are usually recommended for modern bonding agents (fourth-, fifth-, and sixth generation). Bond strengths of fourth-generation bonding agents used with resin composites can be affected by overly dry or overly wet teeth as well as contaminants such as saliva, plasma, zinc oxide–eugenol cement, and non-eugenol zinc oxide cement (Table 3.18) [30]. Re-etching after contamination occurs is effective [30, 31]. Unexpectedly, contamination of enamel with handpiece lubricant when bonded with fourth- and fifth-generation bonding agents does not reduce bond strength [32].

Table 3.18. In vitro tensile bond strengths (MPa) of resin composites used with two fourth-generation bonding agents bonded to human enamel exposed to different contaminants. (From [30])

Etching condition	All-Bond 2	Scotchbond Multipurpose
Air	17.9[c]	19.9[e,f]
Moist	23.1[a]	22.0[e]
Wet	20.6[b]	12.0[g]
Saliva	10.5[d]	12.5[g]
Saliva re-etched	20.5[b]	20.3[e,f]
Plasma	9.9[d]	13.3[g,h]
Plasma re-etched	18.8[b,c]	18.6[f]
ZOE cement	10.0[d]	6.6
ZOE cement re-etched	19.1[b,c]	20.1[e,f]
Non-ZOE cement	5.1	2.4
Non-ZOE cement re-etched	23.1[a]	15.4[h]

The same superscript letter means statistically the same (p=0.05).

Table 3.19. In vitro tensile bond strength (MPa) of resin composite bonded to enamel treated with self-etching bonding agent as a function of etching time and air thinning. (From [33])

Air thinned	Length of application(s)		
	10	20	30
Yes	18.5	20.0	19.3
No	9.9	15.5	15.9

Table 3.20. In vitro microtensile bond strength (MPa) of resin composite bonded to carbamide-peroxide-bleached enamel treated with fifth-generation bonding agents. (From [35])

Condition	Single Bond	Prime & Bond NT
Control	32	33
10% carbamide peroxide	24	24
10% carbamide peroxide, then 10% sodium ascorbate	34	36

Air Thinning

Air thinning can reduce the bond strength of a sixth-generation bonding agent to enamel (Table 3.19) [33].

Chlorhexidine

Chlorhexidine can be applied on the teeth and over orthodontic appliances during treatment to reduce bacterial colonization [34]. Bond strength is not affected if the chlorhexidine is applied after bonding has been completed or as a prophylactic paste on enamel before etching. Bond strength is reduced to an unacceptable level, however, if the chlorhexidine is applied as a layer on etched enamel or on the sealant before the adhesive is applied [34].

Bleaching

Bond strength of resin composite to carbamide-peroxide-bleached teeth treated with fifth-generation bonding agents is reduced, although this reduction apparently can be reversed using sodium ascorbate (Table 3.20) [35].

Bonding to Enamel: In Vivo Studies

Veneers

Strong bonds can be created between porcelain veneers and underlying tooth structure, particularly enamel. A 100% retention rate of porcelain veneers bonded to enamel has been reported over a 5-year period [36].

Pit-and-Fissure Sealants

Pit-and-fissure sealants show a high retention rate over time (Table 3.21), accounting for the caries preventing benefit of this procedure. Even partially sealed teeth may be considerably less susceptible to caries than unsealed teeth [37]. Sealant retention between primary and permanent molars is not statistically different [38]. Topical fluoride treatment applied immediately before placement of sealants does not adversely affect the retention rate [39].

Glass ionomer sealants show decreased retention rates compared with resin-based sealants [47, 55]. Regardless of the anticariogenic effect of this material, the excellent retention of resin-based sealants, which provides a protective physical barrier over caries-susceptible tooth structure, appears more important for caries prevention than the transient benefit of fluoride release over the short time glass ionomer sealants are retained [55–57].

The placement of sealants using rubber dam isolation clearly influenced the retention rate of the sealant in one study [58]; however, other clinical studies evaluating the method of moisture control on sealant quality or retention reveal conflicting results [58]. Attention to detail and perfect isolation for maintenance of a dry field is an important factor in the success of the sealant [55].

Orthodontic Bonding

Orthodontic bonding to enamel has been reviewed in detail [5, 6]. Traditionally, bonding of brackets to enamel has been preceded by etching of the enamel with phosphoric acid, rinsing, and drying, followed by application of an enamel sealant and resin cement. A 5-s etch with phosphoric acid was recently shown to produce a statistically equivalent failure rate when compared clinically with a conventional 15-s etch (Table 3.22) [59].

The use of sixth-generation bonding agents for orthodontic bonding is growing because of the time savings. A clinical study showed a lower failure rate with a self-etching adhesive than conventional etching with phosphoric acid (Table 3.23) [60].

Table 3.21. Retention rates of pit-and-fissure sealants

Observation period (years)	Retention rate (%)	Reference
1	93	[40]
1	94	[41]
1	89, 96[a]	[42]
1	99	[43]
1.5	49	[39]
1.9	63	[44]
2	82	[45]
2	88	[46]
2	97	[43]
3	74	[47]
4	50	[48]
4	73	[46]
4.5	72	[49]
5	42	[37]
5	60	[50]
5	79	[40]
5	82	[51]
6	58	[46]
6	67	[40]
6–7	40	[52]
8–10	41, 85[a]	[42]
10	57	[51]
15	28	[53]
20	65	[54]

[a] Percent total success = percent complete retention + percent partly intact but not requiring resealing + percent which required and received maintenance sealing.

Table 3.22. In vivo failure rate of orthodontic brackets bonded with orthodontic resin cement to enamel using conventional phosphoric acid etching with recommended etch and a 5-s etch. (From [59])

Etching time(s)	Failure rate (%)
15	1.1[a]
5	3.7

[a] Statistically the same (p=0.05).

Table 3.23. In vivo failure rate over 6 months of orthodontic brackets bonded with orthodontic resin cement to enamel using conventional phosphoric acid etching and a self-etching adhesive system. (From [60])

Adhesive system	Failure rate (%)
Phosphoric acid/orthodontic resin cement (Transbond XT)	4.6[a]
Self-etching adhesive (Transbond Plus Self Etching Primer)/ orthodontic resin cement (Transbond XT)	0.6

[a] Statistically different (p=0.05).

References

1. Craig RG, Powers JM, eds. Restorative dental materials, 11th edn. Mosby, St. Louis, 2002
2. Barakat MM, Powers JM. In vitro bond strength of cements to treated teeth. Aust Dent J 1986; 31:415–419
3. Pashley DH, Carvalho RM, Sano H, Nakajima M, Yoshiyama M, Shono Y, Fernandes CA, Tay F. The microtensile bond test: a review. J Adhes Dent 1999; 1:299–309
4. Powers JM, O'Keefe KL, Kaaden C, Pinzon LM. Correlation of inverted cone tensile and microtensile bond strengths. Trans Soc Biomater (CD), vol. 24, 2001
5. Powers JM, Kim H-B, Turner DS. Orthodontic adhesives and bond strength testing. Semin Orthod 1997; 3:147–156
6. Powers JM, Messersmith ML. Enamel etching and bond strength. In: Brantley WA, Eliades T, eds. Orthodontic materials: scientific and clinical aspects. Thieme, New York, 2001, pp 105–122
7. Hobson RS, Mcabe JF, Hogg SD. Bond strength to surface enamel for different tooth types. Dent Mater 2001; 17:184–189
8. Kaaden C, Powers JM, Friedl K-H, Schmalz G. Bond strength of self-etching adhesives to dental hard tissues. Clin Oral Invest 2002; 6:155–160
9. Agostini FG, Kaaden C, Powers JM. Bond strength of self-etching primers to enamel and dentin of primary teeth. Pediatr Dent 2001; 23:481–486
10. Shimada Y, Senawongse P, Harnirattisai C, Burrow MF, Nakaoki Y, Tagami J. Bond strength of two adhesive systems to primary and permanent enamel. Oper Dent 2002; 27:403–409
11. Kanca J III. One Step bond to enamel and dentin. Am J Dent 1997; 9:5–8
12. Swift EJ Jr, Perdigao J, Heymann HO. Enamel bond strengths of "one-bottle" adhesives. Am Acad Pediatr Dent 1998; 20:259–262
13. Hannig M, Reinhardt K-J, Bott B. Self-etching primer vs phosphoric acid: an alternative concept for composite-to-enamel bonding. Oper Dent 1999; 24:172–180
14. Farah JW, Powers JM, eds. Bonding agents. Dent Advis 2002; 19:1–4
15. Tate WH, You C, Powers JM. Bond strength of compomers to human enamel. Oper Dent 2000; 25:283–291
16. Powers JM, Turner DS, Nakano A. Bonding of hybrid ionomers to unetched enamel and orthodontic brackets. Abstr J Dent Res 1996; 75:173
17. Vuu TM, Chang JC, Pinzon LM, Powers JM. Bond strength of self-etching adhesive to human enamel and dentin. Abstr J Dent Res 2003; 82:564
18. Strattman R, Powers JM. Acidic primers utilized to bond orthodontic resins to enamel. Abstr J Dent Res 2001; 80:232
19. Koh SH, You C, Chan JT, Powers JM. Effect of fluoride treatment on bonding of sealants to enamel. Abstr J Dent Res 1997; 76:189
20. Kanemura N, Sano H, Tagami J. Tensile bond strength to and SEM evaluation of ground and intact enamel surfaces. J Dent 1999; 27:523–530

21. Perdigao J, Geraldeli S. Bonding characteristics of self-etching adhesives to intact versus prepared enamel. J Esthet Restor Dent 2003; 15:32–42
22. McGrory KR, Lecrone V, English JD, Powers JM. Bond strengths of orthodontic self-etching primers on ground enamel. Abstr J Dent Res 2003; 82:1195
23. Lecrone V, McGrory KR, English JD, Powers JM. Bond strengths of orthodontic self-etching primers to unground enamel. Abstr J Dent Res 2003; 82:1196
24. Ibarra G, Vargas MA, Armstrong SR, Cobb DS. Microtensile bond strength of self-etching adhesives to ground and unground enamel. J Adhes Dent 2002; 4:115–124
25. Xie J, Flaitz CM, Hicks MJ, Powers JM. Bond strength of composite to caries-like enamel lesions. Abstr J Dent Res 1995; 74:32
26. Roeder LB, Berry EA III, You C, Powers JM. Bond strength of composite to air-abraded enamel and dentin. Oper Dent 1995; 20:186–190
27. Berry EA III, Berry L, Powers JM. Bonding of hybrid ionomer to air-abraded enamel and dentin. Abstr J Dent Res 1994; 73:183
28. Martinez-Insua A, Da Silva DL, Rivera FG, Santana-Penin UA. Differences in bonding to acid-etched or Er:YAG-laser-treated enamel and dentin surfaces. J Prosthet Dent 2000; 84:280–288
29. Trajtenberg CP, Pereira PNR, Powers JM. Resin bond strength and micromorphology of human teeth prepared with an Erbium:YAG laser. Trans Academy of Dental Materials, vol 15. Proc Conference on Scientific Criteria for Selecting Materials and Techniques in Clinical Dentistry, Siena, Italy, 25–27 October 2001, p. 171
30. Xie J, Powers JM, McGuckin RS. In vitro bond strength of two adhesives to enamel and dentin under normal and contaminated conditions. Dent Mater 1993; 9:295–299
31. Powers JM, Finger WJ, Xie J. Bonding of composite resin to contaminated human enamel and dentin. J Prosthodont 1995; 4:28–32
32. Rosa BT, Heymann HO, Swift EJ Jr, Perdigao J, Ritter AV. Shear bond strengths of one-bottle adhesives to oil-contaminated enamel. J Esthet Dent 2000; 12:139–145
33. Shukla BA, Kaaden C, Powers JM. Bond strength sensitivity of self-etching adhesive to application procedure. Abstr J Dent Res 2001; 80:61
34. Bishara SE, Vonwald L, Zamtua J, Damon PL. Effects of various methods of chlorhexidine application on shear bond strength. Am J Orthod Dentofac Orthop 1998; 114:150–153
35. Lai SCN, Tay FR, Cheung GSP, Mak YF, Carvalho RM, Wei SHY, Toledano M, Osorio R, Pashley DH. Reversal of compromised bonding in bleached enamel. J Dent Res 2002; 81: 477–481
36. Peumans M, Van Meerbeek B, Lambrechts P, Vuylsteke-Wauters M, Vanherle G. Five-year clinical performance of porcelain veneers. Quintessence Int 1998; 29:211–221
37. Horowitz HS, Heifetz SB, Poulsen S. Retention and effectiveness of a single application of an adhesive sealant in preventing occlusal caries: final report after five years of a study in Kalispell, Montana. 1977: 95:1133–1139
38. Vrbi V. Retention of a fluoride-containing sealant on primary and permanent teeth 3 years after placement. Quintessence Int 1999; 30:825–828
39. Warren DP, Infante NB, Rice HC, Turner SD, Chan JT. Effect of topical fluoride on retention of pit and fissure sealants. J Dent Hyg 2001; 75:21–24
40. Calderone JJ, Davis JM. The New Mexico sealant program: a progress report. J Public Health Dent 1987; 47:145–149
41. Sterritt GR, Frew RA. Evaluation of a clinic-based sealant program. J Public Health Dent 1988; 48:220–224
42. Romcke RG, Lewis DW, Maze BD, Vickerson RA. Retention and maintenance of fissure sealants over 10 years. J Can Dent Assoc 1990; 56:235–237
43. Whyte RJ, Leake JL, Howley TP. Two-year follow-up of 11,000 dental sealants in first permanent molars in the Saskatchewan Health Dental Plan. J Public Health Dent 1987; 47:177–181
44. Raadal M, Laegreid O, Laegreid KV, Hveem H, Korsgaard EK, Wangen K. Fissure sealing of permanent first molars in children receiving a high standard of prophylactic care Community Dent Oral Epidemiol 1984; 47:145–149
45. Forss H, Saarni U-M, Seppä L. Comparison of glass-ionomer and resin-based fissure sealants: a 2-year clinical trial. Comm Dent Oral Epidemiol 1994; 22:21–24

46. Houpt M, Shey Z. The effectiveness of a fissure sealant after 6 years. Pediatr Dent 1983; 5:104–106
47. Poulsen S, Beiruti N, Sadat N. A comparison of retention and the effect on caries of fissure sealing with a glass-ionomer and a resin-based sealant. Comm Dent Oral Epidemiol 2001; 29:298–301
48. Going RE, Haugh LD, Grainger DA, Conti AJ. Four-year clinical evaluation of a pit and fissure sealant. Am Dent J 1977; 95:972–981
49. Mertz-Fairhurst EJ, Della-Giustina VE, Brooks JE, Williams JE, Fairhurst CW. A comparative study of two pit and fissure sealants: results after 4 years in Augusta, Ga. Am Dent J 1981; 103:235–238
50. Meurman JH, Helminen SK, Luoma H. Caries reduction over 5 years from a single application of a fissure sealant. Scand J Dent Res 1978; 86:153–156
51. Simonsen RJ. Retention and effectiveness of a single application of white sealant after 10 years. Am Dent J 1987; 115:31–36
52. Heidmann J, Poulsen S, Mathiassen F. Evaluation of a fissure sealing programme in a Danish Public Child Dental Service. Comm Dent Health 1990; 7:379–388
53. Simonsen RJ. Retention and effectiveness of dental sealant after 15 years. Am Dent J 1991; 122:34–42
54. Wendt LK, Koch G, Birkhed D. On the retention and effectiveness of fissure sealant in permanent molars after 15–20 years: a cohort study. Comm Dent Oral Epidemiol 2001; 29:302–307
55. Simonsen RJ. Pit and fissure sealant: Review of the literature. Pediatr Dent 2002; 24: 393–414
56. Pereira AC, Basting RT, Pinelli C, de Castro Meneghim M, Werner CW. Retention and caries prevention of Vitremer and Ketac-bond used as occlusal sealants. Am Dent J 1999; 12:62–64
57. Pereira AC, Pardi V, Mialhe FL, Meneghim MC, Basting RT, Werner CW. Clinical evaluation of a polyacid-modified resin used as a fissure sealant. Am Dent J 2000; 13:294–296
58. Ganss C, Klimek J, Gleim A. One-year clinical evaluation of the retention and quality of two fluoride releasing sealants. Clin Oral Invest 1999; 3:188–193
59. Hughes TJ, Kerr SD, Powers JM. Clinical study of the effect of no prophylaxis and reduced etching time on bond strength. J Clin Orthod 2003; 37:99–100
60. Asgari S, Salas A, English J, Powers J. Clinical evaluation of bond failure rates with a new self-etching primer. J Clin Orthod 2002; 36:687–689

Orthodontic Bonding to Wet Enamel with Water-Insensitive and Water-Activated Orthodontic Adhesive Resins

4

T. Eliades, G. Eliades, N. Silikas, D.C. Watts

Introduction

The interference of moisture in enamel bonding procedures is of interest mainly for orthodontic applications and to a lesser extent for bonded restorations. The mechanism and interfacial phenomena of enamel bonding from a restorative dentistry perspective are analyzed in Chap. 1. Also, conventional and resin-modified glass-ionomer cements [1, 2] as well as dentine primers [3] and self-etching primers [4], have been utilized in orthodontic bonding; however, a thorough analysis of the properties and bonding characteristics of these materials with dentine and enamel is provided in the subsequent sections. This scope of this chapter pertains to orthodontic bonding to wet enamel substrate using the recently introduced moisture-insensitive and water-activated polymeric orthodontic adhesives.

In general, the effect of exposure of resinous materials to hydration has been studied for 2–3 decades. In dental composite resins literature, a series of studies have indicated that the effects incurred may affect the matrix, fillers, and filler-matrix bonding, which are discussed later in this chapter.

The inefficiency of adhesive systems in the presence of moisture has long been known through studies showing substantially decreased bond strength for adhesive systems bonded to wet substrates [5]. In recent years, manufacturers have sought to enhance the performance of bonding systems in the presence of moisture by introducing novel materials.

It is noteworthy that the term moist is used to include a wide variety of conditions extending from the presence of water and saliva, to contamination by blood, tissue exudate and crevicular fluid, which are better described as contaminants [5]. Although the presence of water can be prevented by adopting moisture-control precautions during bonding procedures, the orthodontist is often faced with the problem of bonding in an environment with increased contamination risk from saliva [6]. This may be a particular concern in bonding brackets to partially erupted premolars, where the majority of bond failures are usually located [2]. Problems arise because of the proximity of the adhesive to the cervical portion of the crown, the presence of crevicular fluid, the complex and high-magnitude masticatory loads in the posterior dentition, as well as the contour of the crown, which varies substantially for premolars [7].

The products currently available for orthodontic bonding of resins to a wet environment may be classified in moisture-insensitive primers, water-activated adhesives, and hydrophilic resin paste formulations (Table 4.1). Even though these materials possess fundamental differences with respect to their setting mecha-

Table 4.1. Polymerization initiation and compositional characteristics of the adhesives used for bonding in wet environment

Material	Polymerization initiation and application	Compositional characteristics
Smartbond (Gestenco) moisture active	Composite paste formulation only initiation through exposure to water	Cyanoacrylate
Transbond MIP (3 M unitek) hydrophilic monomer	Primer formulation applied to enamel surface	Methacrylate-functionalized polyalkenoic acid copolymer
Assure (Reliance) hydrophilic monomer	Photo-polymerizable paste applied with conventional procedures	Hydrophilic co-monomer

nism or reactivity with moisture, for practicality the aforementioned group of products is referred to as „wet-substrate adhesives" throughout this chapter.

The purpose of this chapter is to summarize the evidence currently available on the effect of moisture and contaminants on the survivorship of the adhesive–enamel bond, to provide evidence to illustrate the source of variability among contradictory bond strength data obtained from studies with respect to nominally identical materials, and to analyze the polymerization mechanism of various adhesives intended for application to wet enamel. Finally, the effect of water and saliva on the structural integrity of composites is discussed.

Approaches in Assessing the Efficiency of Orthodontic Adhesives Systems

Testing of wet-substrate adhesive effectiveness in orthodontics can be classified into two major categories: bond strength studies and clinical-failure-rate protocols. Table 4.2 summarizes the advantages and disadvantages of each protocol.

The Reliability of Bond Strength Testing Protocols

A considerable variability among bond strength studies of same materials is noted probably deriving from the multiplicity of test configurations, as well as the assumptions and approximations integrated in experimental methodologies [7, 8].

It has been found that variability exists among various manufacturers with respect to wing design or dimensions for brackets of a nominally identical prescription [9–10] contributing to the misalignment of loads during testing; thus, the resultant bending moment generated may vary considerably with impact on the stresses developed at the multiple interfaces of the bonding system (enamel–adhesive, adhesive–bracket). This effect can result in substantial differences in the measured force required to cause bond failure [10].

Table 4.2. Classification of research protocols utilized to assess the efficiency of moisture-insensitive adhesives (number in parentheses denote references)

Method	Test/procedure	Comments
Assessment of the bond strength of moisture-insensitive adhesives in the presence of water, saliva, or blood relative to conventional adhesives [2, 4, 8–12]	Mounting on a testing matching and test under shear (most commonly), tensile, or torsional loads of brackets bonded ex vivo to extracted teeth	Advantages: Provides strength values and allows for the study of fractured surfaces to investigate failure pattern Disadvantages: Incorporates many dependent variables including tooth morphological and structural variability, selection, and storage; enamel surface preparation; standardization of wetting by water or saliva; amount of adhesive and force applied on the bracket; specimen mounting and testing [45]. These problems coupled with the notable lack of a clinically derived minimum requirement for bond strength threshold make the clinical relevance of the method problematic. Also, the involvement of masticatory forces and aging of adhesive cannot be assessed and thus no information on long-term bond survival can be extrapolated [6]. Analysis of data either by comparison of means or Weibull analysis may also differentiate results.
Clinical failure rate of brackets bonded to enamel with various adhesives over a period of 6–12 months [1, 2]	Number/percent of debonded brackets during orthodontic treatment for various adhesive groups	Advantages: Clinically relevant method (the studied variable is the actual survival of bonds) Disadvantages: It does not provide insight into the cause and pattern of failure; no information on the mechanism of polymerization; difficult to apply in an office setup; requires large clinical environment but in this case a meticulous design is necessary to avoid cross-effects from other confounding individual-related (habits, masticatory forces) or operator-induced (mechanics, handling, bonding procedures) variables
Study of the polymerization reaction of moisture-insensitive adhesives [4]	Study of the degree of cure (IR spectroscopy)	Advantages: Provides evidence of polymerization mechanism and chemical configuration allowing understanding of the phenomena occurring during bonding Disadvantages: No information on mechanical properties or clinical survival rate

Additional several important factors, which may vary among studies, include the method of load application, e.g., tension, shear/peel or torsion, and the crosshead speed of the testing machine, which is typically set at 1 mm/min but may range from 1 to 10 mm/min. The effect of the latter may be twofold: first various investigations have utilized different loading rates ranging from 1 to 10 mm/min with a notable impact on the comparability of the results. In addition, the reliability in simulating the strength of appliances during mastication and the occasional contact of brackets with opposing teeth may be questioned since the standard rates employed in the literature are irrelevant to the velocity of teeth occluding during chewing. A complete masticatory cycle (sequential opening and closing) of a healthy individual lasts approximately 800 ms with the closing movement having a duration less than 400 ms, considering that the movement on biting is accelerated [11]. This figure may be translated roughly to 2000 mm/min, a value substantially higher compared with the standard 1 mm/min rate employed in conventional bond strength protocols. This value remains unaffected by the hardness of bolus setting the integrity of bond at risk [12], because high loading rates eliminate the viscoelastic response of the polymeric adhesive to the applied load, inducing a stiff body response [13], which decreases bond strength [14].

The results of bond strength testing should be expressed in force units (N) as opposed to pressure units (Pa) since the transformation of force to pressure requires the estimation of the actual surface contact area, which cannot be approximated by the surface area of the rectangular base because of the base mesh design patterns [8]. In addition, dividing the force values by the base surface area to estimate the pressure values, implies that the distribution of the load applied is homogeneous across the entire bracket base, a hypothesis which was proved to be erroneous [10].

Finally, the analysis of data employing either comparison of bond strength mean values or Weibull analysis may yield different results for identical strength values. This is because the latter method takes into account the distribution of values as opposed to comparison of a single value (mean) [8, 9, 15].

The influence of the foregoing parameters on the comparability of the results of bond strength studies has been illustrated by Fox and associates who reviewed 60 publications concerning the bond strength of a very common chemically cured adhesive. It was concluded that variations during various steps of testing precluded a reliable extrapolation of a consensus concerning its performance [8].

The Clinical Relevance of Bond Strength Testing

In addition to the practical problems and standardization difficulties encountered in bond strength testing, a concern has developed during recent years about the actual clinical relevance of ex vivo bond strength protocols. Some authors have proposed that these studies fail to simulate the multi-factorial intraoral aging of resin composites [16], which include pH fluctuation, complex cyclic loading, microbial attack, and enzymatic degradation (discussed later). All these factors have been known to induce a plasticizing effect on the material, which adversely affects the mechanical properties and resistance to solubility of composite resins. The series of effects accompanying the intraoral aging of the material may not be reflected on the short-term bond strength performance of the adhesive because bond strength as a variable is not a reliable estimate of the polymerization efficiency and associated properties such as solubility, which may impact the long-term survival of the bond [17–18].

How Much Strength is Required Clinically?

An interesting issue which has caused a turmoil in the relevant orthodontic materials literature pertains to the actual clinical requirement of bond strength based on the estimation of the magnitude of forces developed during orthodontic treatment by the activated archwires. Most studies refer to a 1970s paper by Reynolds [19] who proposed a value of 6–8 MPa, based on the loads developed during archwire engagement in the bracket slot. This number has been cited more than 150 times in the literature as the minimum requirement for a clinically derived bond strength threshold value.

However, this proposition is outdated and depends largely on the mechanics and materials and the overall clinical procedures at the time of its introduction, approximately 30 years ago. It is also conjectural since it is based on a vague assumed load application during mechanotherapy and presents an undefined margin of safety. Also, the proposed value does not take into account the stresses developed during mastication and associated loads developed during chewing hard food at high velocities. Moreover, the foregoing discussion on the intraoral aging of adhesive resins has indicated that intraorally, polymeric adhesives are subjected to cyclic fatigue [20], extreme pH and temperature variations, microbial degradation [21], and are exposed to water, saliva, acidic beverages, and alcohol-containing liquids, which decrease the glass transition temperature of the material, inducing a plasticizing effect [22]; therefore, „threshold strengths" may not cover the requirements for a sound bond throughout the entire period of treatment, which may exceed 18 months. This fact receives greater interest when the lack of comparison of the magnitude of in vitro and in vivo loads is considered [23].

Lastly, there is a trend in the relevant literature to compare the values derived from bond strength data to the aforementioned conjectural threshold value, especially when the bond strength of the experimental product is lower than its standard bonding counterpart [4, 24, 25]. This notion caries two fundamental flaws: first the efficiency of an experimental product should be tested against the performance of a typical, routinely used application and not to anecdotal evidence, which is based on the proposition of one study in the 1970s. Moreover, the comparison of the values obtained from a testing procedure with that of a given standard requires the statistical analysis in the form of a paired *t*-test and cannot be performed by arbitrarily weighing the two mean values. In general, bond strength data interpretation should be limited to relative effectiveness of different adhesives, and thus the tactic of extrapolating absolute values and comparing them with a vaguely defined gold standard should be avoided.

Clinical Bracket Failure Rate

Clinical bond failure has become very popular recently because of its profound clinical relevance associated with the fact that the independent variable is the actual survival of bonds; however, this method does not provide an insight into the cause and pattern of failure and reveals no information on the mechanism of polymerization and site of failure. Moreover, this protocol is very demanding from a setup perspective, since it is difficult to apply in an ordinary office setup and usually requires large clinical environments such as those found in educational institutions. In that case, this method presents some complexities arising from the intervention of multiple operators, the requirement for a meticulous design involving selection of participants who seek treatment in an academic institution with respect to their socio-economic status, and the need for special bonding schemes, i.e., split-mouth pattern. These precautions aim at avoiding cross-effects from other confounding variables including those participant-related (habits, masticatory forces which vary with facial type, diet), or operator-induced (mechanics, handling of materials, bonding procedures). Differences in failure rates noted between males and females [26] possibly attributed to the higher masticatory forces of the former, as well as contradictory evidence derived from studies testing identical materials in different countries or populations, imply that culturally influenced dietary habits and sex differences may modulate the failure rate of brackets in vivo.

Wet-Enamel Adhesives

While some manufacturers claim acceptable performance for their moisture-insensitive or hydrophilic products in a wet environment, others have introduced moisture-active adhesives [26].

The moisture-insensitive adhesive (MIP-3 M/Unitek) is available in a primer formulation that replaces the conventional bonding agents. It is applied to the enamel surface and consists of an aqueous solution of methacrylate-functionalized polyalkenoic acid copolymer and hydroxyethyl-methacrylate. This product has been originally used as a hydrophilic primer in dentine bonding systems marketed by the same manufacturer.

Also, a hydrophilic monomer-based light-cured paste formulation has been introduced by the industry as an alternative adhesive, which requires no additional primer or procedure.

Finally, in contrast to the moisture-insensitive primer, water-activated adhesives require the presence of moisture to induce polymerization initiation. The moisture-active adhesive represents a distinct material available as a cyanoacrylate-based paste formulation, applied to intentionally wetted etched enamel without the use of a primer [6].

Structure and Reactivity with Water

Spectroscopic studies [5] showed that the moisture-insensitive primer and adhesive tested demonstrate completely different reactivity with water. In Transbond MIP, water induces partial ionization of carboxyl groups, and an inert dilution effect without activating any setting mechanism. On the contrary, in Smartbond water initiates a setting mechanism via nucleophilic attack to isocyanate groups leading to a polyurethane film formation. This is a key difference in understanding the bonding mechanisms involved and the interfacial performance of these products in bond strength testing.

Figure 4.1 illustrates the FTIR spectrum of Transbond MIP before and after water application. Water exposure induces an increase in the intensity of the hydrogen-bonded O-H vibrations (3500–3250 cm^{-1} stretching and 1642 cm^{-1} bending); however, the intensity of the hydrogen-bonded unionized carboxyl dimer vibrations (2700–2500 cm^{-1} stretching) was reduced and the complex ester peak (1720 cm^{-1}) was shifted to lower frequency due to partial ionization of carboxyl groups. No differences were observed in the relative intensity of C=C stretching vibrations (1638 cm^{-1}) of the methacrylate moieties, which are related to free-radical polymerization with the primer state remaining liquid.

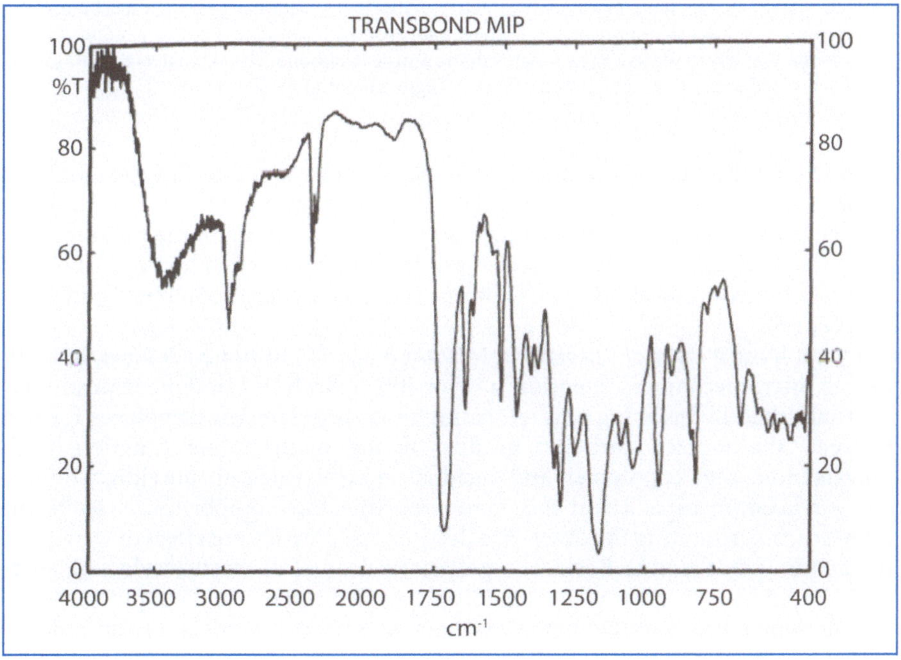

Fig. 4.1. The FTIR spectra of a moisture-insensitive primer (Transbond MIP), which is based on a methacrylate-functionalized polycarboxylic component, shows a characteristic broad band over the 2750–2500 cm^{-1} region due to the formation of H-bonded carboxylic dimers

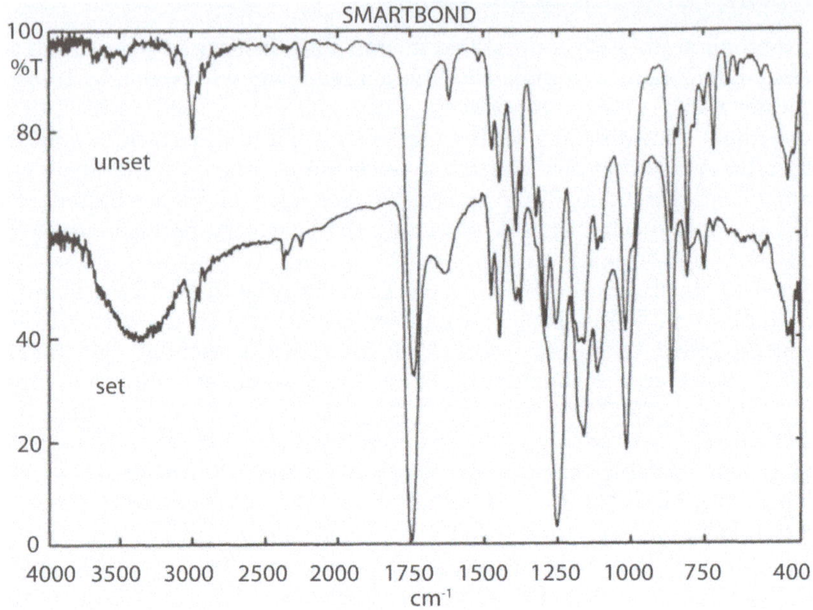

Fig. 4.2. The FTIR spectrum of a moisture-active orthodontic adhesive (Smartbond) before and after setting. The intensity of the original isocyanate group (NCO^- at 2239 cm^{-1}) is reduced in the set film due to the formation on the polyurethane amide backbone. The set material contains hydrogen-bonded water (OH^- at 3400 cm^{-1}) and a high content of CO_2 (2364 cm^{-1})

In Fig. 4.2 the FTIR spectrum of Smartbond before and after water addition is shown. The intensity of the original isocyanate group (NCO stretching at 2239 cm^{-1}) was reduced in the set film due to the formation on the polyurethane amide backbone. The adhesive was set producing a film rich in hydrogen-bonded water (O-H stretching at 3400 cm^{-1}), amine (N-H stretching at 3300 cm^{-1}), and CO_2 (2364 cm^{-1}).

By applying a layer of Transbond MIP onto acid-conditioned enamel, in addition to micromechanical retention, a reversible hydrolytic bond mechanism may be established by breaking and reforming of carboxylate salt complexes formed between the ionized carboxyl groups of the methacrylate functionalized-polyalkenoic acid copolymer and residual enamel calcium, providing limited stress-relaxation capacity. In this manner, a dynamic equilibrium is set at the interface, incorporating the otherwise detrimental plasticizing effect of water, into the bonding mechanism. Besides, copolymerization of the methacrylate moieties of the copolymer with the resin is mediated by the presence of the rapid-responding monomer hydroxyethylmethacrylate. This may counterbalance the reduced extent of conversion of the methacrylate groups attached to the high molecular weight polyalkenoic acid copolymer caused by steric hindrance [28, 29].

The application of primer may be problematic in combination with dual-paste and no-mix adhesives. In the latter systems, setting of these materials involves the diffusion of the liquid resin brushed on bracket base and enamel surface into the paste through the application of pressure during bracket placement. Therefore, from a structural and setting mechanism it seems that the application of Transbond MIP may not be compatible with the orthodontic adhesive pastes.

The performance of the hydrophilic primer may be associated with its highly hydrophilic nature along with its participation in two interfaces possessing dissimilar characteristics. The presence of a hydrophilic factor may allow for improved wetting of etched enamel and possibly involvement of the stress relaxation bonding mechanism discussed above; however, the interface with the adhesive paste seems to be disturbed due to incompatibility between the hydrophilic primer and the hydrophobic adhesive resin. This may result in poor diffusion of the liquid primer into the adhesive paste and inadequate copolymerization. Moreover, the acidic nature of the primer may protonize the amine component of the chemically cured systems thereby reducing the amine activation capacity. The increased frequency of resin adhesive failures observed in Transbond MIP treated groups in associated studies supports such a mechanism [14].

The original dentine bonding system, where a primer similar to Transbond MIP was introduced, incorporated the additional step of bonding resin placement prior to composite application in the chemically cured systems. This resin consisted of a mixture of hydrophilic and hydrophobic monomers, i.e., bis-GMA and HEMA to improve the compatibility of its constituents; thus, intermixing of the primer and bonding resin components in situ facilitated homogeneity of free radical production and effective copolymerization of the primer and bonding resin components; however, this may not be achieved with a no-mix system, where intermixing of the components seems difficult due to monomer incompatibility and viscosity difference. A potential improvement could involve intermixing of Transbond MIP and adhesive primer before application to etched enamel surface.

Smartbond is a single-phase, particle-filled adhesive based on cyanoacrylate chemistry, which sets in the presence of water and this may be considered as an inherent advantage of the material. The setting reaction of this product involves two steps. In the first step isocyanate groups react with water, forming an unstable carbamic acid component, which rapidly decomposes to carbon dioxide and the corresponding amine. In the second step the amine reacts with residual isocyanate groups, crosslinking the adhesive through substituted urea groups [30]; however, in the presence of excess water, the first step of the reaction, namely the formation of amine and carbon dioxide, is enhanced, resulting in reduced film-fracture toughness [27].

An additional problem with these systems relates to the release of carbon dioxide which is only capable of limited diffusion through the adhesive film. As polymerization proceeds, it may become entrapped, forming gaps or voids with possible detrimental effects on the interfacial strength [31], as analyzed below. This hypothesis is supported by the increased frequency of cohesive failures found for the Smartbond adhesive implying the development of reduced network connectivity and bulk discontinuities due to void inclusion [6].

Ex vivo and Laboratory Performance

Interestingly, the chemical structure and physical properties of the materials intended for use in the wet environment and their reactivity with moisture have received limited attention with only one paper reporting on the polymerization reaction of the materials [6]. Considering the vast amount of interactions of many confounding variables during testing and the foregoing parameters, which interfere with strength data analysis [32], it seems that the investigators focused on the performance of the systems, without having a clear picture of the structure and polymerization efficiency of these materials.

The effectiveness of adhesives, which can be used in moist environments, has been the objective of a relatively large number of studies, which approached the subject mostly from the bond strength aspect of testing; thus, a number of papers present evidence of comparative bond strength results of moisture-insensitive primer or paste formulations and standard bonding protocols. It seems that the only point of agreement among these studies is the detrimental effect of moisture on conventional bonding protocols, which show a considerable decrease in bond strength [3, 22, 33]. The literature is inconclusive with respect to the effectiveness of wet-substrate adhesives, owing to the implication of variables analyzed in the previous section.

Thus, whereas a group of investigations have shown that bond strength data for the hydrophilic primer showed superior or comparable results to that of conventional bonding materials [34], other laboratory studies suggested the opposite [6, 15, 35]. The results of the studies support the proposition to use this primer only with light-cured adhesive systems since its application with one- or two-phase adhesives presumably interferes with the setting reaction of the adhesive producing poor strength [6, 35].

The hydrophilic adhesive paste formulation has generally shown decreased bond strength [34] and higher failure rate [36] relative to the moisture-insensitive primer.

Lastly, the body of the literature on the performance of the moisture-active adhesive shows a dispute over its performance. Whilst some studies find the bond strength acceptable [5], other laboratory investigations report poor performance [6], whereas clinical failure rate studies indicate an increased frequency of debonded brackets [37].

Effect of Water and Contaminants on Orthodontic Adhesive Resins

Hydration and contaminants in the form of saliva, crevicular fluid, or blood have potent effects on both elements of bonding: substrate and material. Their effects on etched enamel have long been well known as irreversible adsorption of the honeycomb enamel pattern. Whereas the long-term influence of these factors on the composite resin structure has been shown to involve swelling and solubility, little evidence is available on their short-term effects.

The detrimental effect of moisture on orthodontic resin adhesives pertains to water adsorption and exertion of a plasticizing effect in the polymer network from the creation of hydrated zones at polar monomer sites. In addition, oxidation of pendant C=C bonds attached to the network, which release by-products such as formaldehyde, may have a pronounced plasticizing effect [38].

The majority of the evidence currently available on the hydrolytic degradation of resin composites derives from the studies by Söderholm and colleagues who have thoroughly investigated the effect of hydration on matrix, fillers, and filler-matrix bonding [39–44]. (For a thorough analysis of the effect of water on the material, the reader is referred to the chapter „In vivo degradation mechanisms of dental resin composites“ by Söderholm [45]).

Effect of Hydration on Resin Matrix

Water sorption by matrix is considered the first step in a sequence of events leading to plasticizing of the polymer and a notable reduction of its mechanical properties and physical characteristics. In general, degradation of the resin matrix depends largely on the degree of C=C conversion as a sufficiently polymerized polymer increases the network density minimizing solubility, as well as diffusion of water through the matrix. This may minimize the release of monomers and various amines such as polymerization accelerators and initiators with proven cytotoxicity [46].

In analyzing the effect of hydration on polymer, it is important to consider that the set polymeric adhesive contains carbon atoms at three different binding states:

1. Converted double bonds forming the crosslinked network
2. Unreacted C=C bonds (remaining monomer)
3. Unreacted C=C bonds attached to the crosslinked network (pendant)

The potent effect of water in the form of hydration is concerned mainly with the last two categories. The development of a network in the presence of water involves the absorption of water molecules, which may cause swelling and structural defects. This gives rise to release of unreacted groups in the form of residual monomer, with pronounced effects on the mechanical profile and biological behavior of the material.

Water also forms hydrogen bonding with MMA group and ether chain linkages of the dimethacrylate monomers that they may interfere with the conversion capacity of C=C.

Effect of Hydration on Fillers and Filler–Matrix Interface

Water can cause hydrolytic breakdown of the filler surface through either elemental leaching from the filler surface or destruction of the filler-matrix bonding.

Water molecules diffused into the matrix can attack the glass (silica, alumina) filler surface causing breakdown. This effect is due to the replacement of leached filler-contained sodium by hydrogen, which takes place because of the smaller size of the latter ion. This effect induces tensile stresses on the outer layer of the glass, which lead to stress corrosion. Each one of the absorbed hydrogen leaves its correspondent OH^- ion free, causing a rise in the pH. Upon exceeding a critical value of acidity, OH^- ions induce rupturing the siloxane bonds of the silanated glass surface, leading to failure of the glass surface.

This mechanism was first described by Söderholm and associates to occur in a glass-filled poly(methylmethacrylate) model material simulating a dental resin composite and later similar degradation mechanisms were identified for dental resin composites.

It is noteworthy that storage of resin composite materials in a saliva-simulating solution induces higher filler leaching relative to that obtained from identical materials stored in distilled water, apparently due to the effect of different ions at the interface [43].

Other factors implicated in filler degradation have been shown to include fluoride compounds, especially in the from of topical acidulated phosphate fluoride (APF) [47], which cause extensive loss of filler from the composite specimens, relative to standard NaF solutions [48].

The filler–silane–resin complex interface may degrade as well, because of the outer filler surface degradation. This induces stress-transfer phenomena, which detach the coupling agent from the filler surface, causing complete debonding. Sharp filler particles tend to present increased stress concentration localized to edges which results in crack growth and failure of the filler-matrix bond. In contrast, spherical-shaped micro-fillers cause less stress-raising effect because of their shape, reducing leaching.

An additional failure mechanism could be enzymatic degradation of the silane molecule covering the fillers [49]. The effect of enzymes on solubility and degradation of composites is discussed later.

Hydrolysis and Degradation of Composite Resins

Degradation of composite resins is coupled with two major biocompatibility concerns: the first is the release of residual monomer, which has been implicated in toxicity and allergic reactions. The extent of release depends on the potency of the environment or immersion media of composites. The second concern is the release of formaldehyde resulting from the oxidation of pendant C=C. It has been shown that formaldehyde released from the composite surface could be detected even after 4 months of immersion in water [45]. The formation of formaldehyde may be increased with increasing oxygen inhibition of the polymerizations reaction. This undesirable effect is present mainly in the two-phase systems where the prolonged reaction is further enhanced by the mixing of the paste and liquid components of the adhesives. This process forms voids and entrapping air in the material, increasing the porosity and inhibition of the reaction [27].

Also, localized bacteria and enzymes may then penetrate the surface of the resin and accelerate the degradation process. Since a definite link between water sorption, solubility, and polymerization exists, increased monomer concentration and carbon double-bond unsaturation might predispose the material to potent degradation reactions. Evidence of the detrimental effects of enzymes and enzyme metabolism by-products on dental resin surfaces has been presented in the literature. Munksgaard and Freud demonstrated the occurrence of enzyme-induced degradation of dimethacrylate polymers and the hydrolytic nature of the process [50, 51]. Their work was succeeded by experiments in several polymer systems that consistently showed enzymatic activity-induced degradation of the materials [52]. Initially, the applicability of these laboratory results to the clinical situation was questioned on the basis of the formation of a proteinaceous film intraorally covering the material surface.

Enzymes, such as esterase, normally present in the oral cavity were found capable of hydrolyzing the polymer by breaking the ester linkages found in different resins. The resistance of composite resins to esterase-induced softening may be dependent on the molecular weight of the monomer since high molecular weight monomer molecules, such as the bis-GMA, present higher resistance than monomers of decreased molecular weight such as the TEGDMA [45].

Matasa has also demonstrated the microbial degradation of composites by providing evidence of aerobic and anaerobic microbial attack of adhesives attached to debonded brackets [21]. The action of these micro-organisms, which can metabolize resin constituents, may weaken the resin, leading to compromised bond strength. A suggestion was made to incorporate substances in the adhesive with bactericidal activity, similar to the approach of including gentamycin in bone cements intended for use in total hip replacement arthroplasties; however, no documented evidence regarding the feasibility of introducing such a product is currently available.

The effect of saliva on the alteration of polymeric material properties has not been investigated in the broader dental materials literature. It could be postulated that the presence of a high mucous protein content and enzymes would result in increased degradation reactions in the adhesive. While enzymatic degradation of dental polymers has been shown previously, no documented evidence exists regarding saliva-induced alterations. Since material degradation reactions constitute a long-term process, their results may be masked by the immediate and more invasive action of water on the polymer structure.

Lastly, the effect of blood has been described to induce sharp decline in the bond strength of conventional adhesives [53], although others found no effect of contamination [54]. Further evidence is required to resolve the dispute which can be attributed to non-standardized testing protocols.

References

1. Cacciafesta V, Jost-Brinkman PG, Süssenberger U, Miethke RR. Effects of saliva and water contamination on the enamel shear bond strength of a light-cured glass ionomer cement. Am J Orthod Dentofac Orthop 1998; 113:402–407
2. Cacciafesta V, Bosch C, Melsen B. Clinical comparison between a resin-reinforced self-cured glass ionomer cement and a composite resin for direct bonding of orthodontic brackets. Part 1: Wetting with water. Clin Orthod Res 1998; 1:29–36
3. Jain P, Stewart GP. Effect of dentin primer on shear bond strength of composite resin to moist and dry enamel. Oper Dent 2000; 25:51–58
4. Cacciafesta V, Sfondrini MF, Angelis M de, Scribante A, Klersy C. Effect of water and saliva contamination on shear bond strength of brackets bonded with conventional, hydrophilic, and self-etching primers. Am J Orthod Dentofacial Orthop 2003; 123:633–640
5. Bishara SE, Wald L von, Laffoon JF, Warren JJ. Effect of using a new cyanoacrylate adhesive on the shear bond strength of orthodontic brackets. Angle Orthod 2001; 71:466–469
6. Eliades T, Katsavrias E, Eliades G. Moisture-insensitive adhesives: reactivity with water and bond strength to wet and saliva-contaminated enamel. Eur J Orthod 2002; 24:35–42

7. Eliades T, Brantley WA. The inappropriateness of conventional orthodontic bond strength assessment protocols. Eur J Orthod 2000; 22:13–23
8. Fox NA, McCabe JF, Buckley JG. A critique of bond strength testing in orthodontics. Br J Orthod 1994; 21:33–43
9. Katona TR, Chen J. Engineering and experimental analyses of the tensile loads applied during strength testing of direct bonded orthodontic brackets. Am J Orthod Dentofac Orthop 1994; 106:167–174
10. Katona TR, Moore BK. The effects of load misalignment on tensile load testing of direct bonded orthodontic brackets: a finite element model. Am J Orthod Dentofac Orthop 1994; 105:543–551
11. Buschang PH, Hayasaki H, Throckmorton GS. Quantification of human chewing-cycle kinematics. Arch Oral Biol 2000 45:461–474
12. Anderson K, Throckmorton GS, Buschang PH, Havasaki H. The effects of bolus hardness on masticatory kinematics. J Oral Rehabil 2002; 29:689–696
13. Braem M, Davidson CL, Vanherle G, van Doren V, Lambrechts P. The relationship between test methodology and elastic behavior of composites. J Dent Res 1987; 5:1036–1039
14. Eliades T, Katsavrias E, Zinelis S, Eliades G. Effect of loading rate on bond strength of brackets bonded to enamel. J Orofac Orthop 2004; 65:336–342
15. Littlewood SJ, Mitchell L, Greenwood DC, Bubb NL, Wood DJ. Investigation of a hydrophylic primer for orthodontic bonding: an in vitro study. J Orthod 2000; 27:181–186
16. Eliades T. Comparing bond strengths (Letter). Am J Orthod Dentofacial Orthop 2002; 122:13A–15A
17. Eliades T, Eliades G, Brantley WA, Johnston WM. Polymerization efficiency of chemically cured and visible light-cured orthodontic adhesives: degree of cure. Am J Orthod Dentofacial Orthop 1995; 108:294–301
18. Eliades T, Eliades G, Brantley WA, Johnston WM. Monomer leaching from chemically cured and visible light-cured orthodontic adhesives. Am J Orthod Dentofacial Orthop 1995; 108:316–321
19. Reynolds. A review of direct orthodontic bonding. Br J Orthod 1975; 2:171–178
20. Moseley HC, Horrocks EN, Pearson GJ, Davies EH. Effects of cyclic stressing on attachment bond strength using glass ionomer cement and composite resin. Br J Orthod 1995; 22:23–27
21. Matasa CG. Microbial attack of orthodontic adhesives. Am J Orthod Dentofacial Orthop 1995; 108:132–141
22. Hobson RS, McCabe JF, Hogg SD. The effect of food simulants on enamel-composite bond strength. J Orthod. 2000; 27:55–59
23. Murray SD, Hobson RS. Comparison of in vivo and in vitro shear bond strength. Am J Orthod Dentofacial Orthop 2003; 123:2–9
24. Bishara SE, Wald L von, Laffoon JF, Warren JJ. Effect of using a new cyanoacrylate adhesive on the shear bond strength of orthodontic brackets. Angle Orthod 2001; 71:466–469
25. Haydar B, Sarikaya S, Cehreli ZC. Comparison of shear bond strength of three bonding agents with metal and ceramic brackets. Angle Orthod 1999; 69:457–462
26. Adolfsson U, Larsson E, Ogaard B. Bond failure of a no-mix adhesive during orthodontic treatment. Am J Orthod Dentofacial Orthop 2002; 122:277–281
27. Eliades T, Eliades G. Orthodontic adhesive resins. In: Brantley W A, Eliades T, eds. Orthodontic materials: scientific and clinical aspects. Thieme, Stuttgart, 2001, pp 201–21
28. Eliades G. Clinical relevance of the formulation and testing of dentin bonding systems. J Dent 1994; 22:73–81
29. Peters WJ, Jackson RW, Smith DC. Studies of the stability and toxicity of zinc polyacrylate (polycarboxylate)cements (PAZ). J Biomed Mater Res 1974; 8:53–60
30. Turner GPA. Introduction to paint chemistry and principles of paint technology, Chapman and Hall, London, 1980
31. Korbmacher H, Klocke A, Huck L, Kahl-Nieke B. Evaluation of a new one-phase orthodontic adhesive. Eur J Orthod 2000; 22:595 (Abstract)

32. Brantley WA, Eliades T, Litsky AS. Mechanics and mechanical testing of orthodontic materials. In: Brantley WA, Eliades T (eds) Orthodontic materials: scientific and clinical aspects. Thieme, Stuttgart, 2001, pp 27–49
33. Webster MJ, Nanda RS, Duncanson MG Jr, Khajotia SS, Sinha PK. The effect of saliva on shear bond strengths of hydrophilic bonding systems. Am J Orthod Dentofacial Orthop 2001; 119:54–58
34. Schaneveldt S, Foley TF. Bond strength comparison of moisture-insensitive primers. Am J Orthod Dentofacial Orthop 2002; 12:267–273
35. Grandhi RK, Combe EC, Speidel TM. Shear bond strength of stainless steel orthodontic brackets with a moisture-insensitive primer. Am J Orthod Dentofacial Orthop 2001; 119:251–255
36. Mavropoulos A, Karamouzos A, Kolokithas G, Athanasiou AE. In vivo evaluation of two moisture-resistant orthodontic adhesive systems: a comparative clinical trial: J Orthod 2003; 30:139–147
37. Karamouzos A, Mavropoulos A, Athanasiou AE, Kolokithas G. In vivo evaluation of a moisture-activated orthodontic adhesive: a comparative clinical trial. Orthod Craniofac Res 2002; 5:170–178
38. Cook WD. Polymerization defects in composite resins. In: Vanherle G, Smith DC, eds. Posterior composite resin dental restorative materials. Peter Szulc, The Netherlands, 1984
39. Söderholm KJ. Degradation of glass filler in experimental composites. J Dent Res 1981; 60:1867
40. Söderholm K-J, Zigan M, Ragan M, Fischlschweiger W, Bergman M. Hydrolytic degradation of dental composites. J Dent Res 1984; 63:1248
41. Söderholm K-J. Leaking of fillers in dental composites. J Dent Res 1993; 62:126
42. Söderholm, K-J. Filler systems and resin interface. In: Vanherle G, Smith DC, eds. Posterior composite resin dental restorative materials. Peter Szulc, Utrecht, The Netherlands, 1984, p 139
43. Söderholm K-J. Filler leachability during water storage of six composite materials. Scand J Dent Res 1990; 98:82
44. Söderholm K-J, Mukherjee R, Longmate J. Filler leachability of composites stored in distilled water or artificial saliva. J Dent Res 1996; 75:1692
45. Söderholm K-J. In vivo degradation mechanisms of dental resin composites. In: Eliades G, Eliades T, Brantley WA, Watts DC, eds. Dental materials in vivo: aging and related phenomena. Quintessence, Chicago, 2003, pp 99–125
46. Eliades T, Eliades G, Bradley TG, Watts DC. Degree of cure of orthodontic adhesives with various polymerization initiation modes. Eur J Orthod 2000; 22:395–399
47. Papagiannoulis L, Tzoutzas J, Eliades G. Effect of topical fluoride agents on the morphologic characteristics and composition of resin composite restorative materials. J Prosthet Dent 1997; 77:405
48. Kula K, McKinney JE, Kula TJ. Effects of daily topical fluoride gels on resin degradation and wear. Dent Mater 1997; 13:305
49. Billmeyer FW Jr (ed) Thermosetting resins. In: Textbook of polymer science. Wiley, New York, 1984, pp 436–457
50. Munksgaard EC, Freud M. Enzymatic hydrolysis of (di)methacrylates and their polymers. Scand J Dent Res 1990; 98:261
51. Freud M, Munksgaard EC. Enzymatic degradation of Bis-GMA/TEGDMA polymers causing decreased microhardness and greater wear in vitro. Scand J Dent Res 1990; 98:351–355
52. de Gee AJ, Wendt SL, Werner A, Davidson CL. Influence of enzymes and plaque acids on in vitro wear of dental composites. Biomaterials 1996; 17:1327
53. Oonsombat C, Bishara SE, Ajlouni R. The effect of blood contamination on the shear bond strength of orthodontic brackets with the use of a new self etch primer. Am J Orthod Dentofacial Orthop 2003; 123:547–550
54. Reddy L, Marker VA, Ellis E III. Bond strength for orthodontic brackets contaminated by blood: composite versus resin-modified glass ionomer cements. J Oral Maxillofac Surg. 2003; 61:206–213

Part II
Bonding to Dentine

Bonding to Dentin: Smear Layer and the Process of Hybridization

5

K. Van Landuyt, J. De Munck, E. Coutinho, M. Peumans, P. Lambrechts, B. Van Meerbeek

Introduction

The use of composite filling materials along with adhesive techniques has revolutionized present dental practice. The esthetic potential, handling, and wear properties of composite fillings have improved drastically [1]. In the hands of a skilled dentist, composite fillings are able to replace lost tooth tissue in an invisible way; however, no matter how splendid the shape and color, a good composite filling does not last long without good bonding to the remaining tooth structure.

Whereas amalgam fillings have no other retention than the cavity in which they are placed, composite fillings can be "glued" to enamel and dentin with an adhesive, thereby permitting a less invasive restorative therapy. Obviously, this bonding is of primordial importance because of the chewing forces a composite filling needs to withstand. In addition, a good adhesive should be able to prevent leakage along the restoration's margins. Clinically, failure of a composite filling occurs more often due to inadequate sealing, with subsequent discoloration of the cavity margins, than to loss of retention [2, 3].

Basically, the main bonding mechanism of current adhesives can be regarded as an exchange process involving substitution of inorganic tooth material by resin monomers that upon in situ setting become micromechanically interlocked in the created microporosities [4]. Diffusion is the primary mechanism to obtain such micromechanical retention. Recently, more evidence has corroborated a possible and additional bonding mechanism, i.e., chemical bonding between specific monomers and calcium in hydroxyapatite [5].

Many factors relating to the adhesive itself and the bonding substrate influence the adhesive performance. In general, bonding to dentin is more challenging than to enamel, because of the complex and hydrated structure of dentin. Dentin is an intricate bonding substrate, and in order to obtain good bonding to dentin an extended knowledge of the structure and composition of the bonding substrate is indispensable. Whereas enamel makes a uniform bonding substrate that consists of almost 90 vol% inorganic material with a very small amount of intrinsic water, dentin is a complex composite material with less than 50 vol% inorganic material, and with high water content (21 vol%). Moreover, the tubular build-up of dentin and the resulting outward pulpal water current in vital teeth turn dentin into a complex substrate. In addition, the effect of tooth type [6], the bonding location (deep vs superficial dentin, crown vs root dentin) [7–11], and tooth qualities (young, old, sclerotic dentin) [12–15] on adhesion receptiveness must be taken into account. In practice, however, dentists will never come across an untouched dentin surface to bond to, since the cavity preparation technique seriously affects the upper layer of dentin.

The first part of this chapter deals with the various forms of smear layers produced by different cavity preparation tools. In the second part, the process of hybridization is described and analyzed. Adhesives categorized according to a standard classification are discussed, and their mechanism of adhesion to dentin is illustrated by diverse microscopy images.

Dentin Substrate: Smear Layer

Cavity preparation alters the uppermost layer of tooth tissue. Research has confirmed that the resultant dentin surface for bonding depends on the preparation technique employed [16, 17].

Nowadays, different instrumentation techniques can be applied to remove caries and to make the tooth surface receptive for bonding. Drilling with a diamond or tungsten carbide bur is the most common way of cavity preparation, but recently more research has been carried out on alternative means of preparing tooth tissue. Bur preparation of cavities often leads to more extensive cavities as compared with the initial caries lesions. Moreover, approximal beveling of cavities

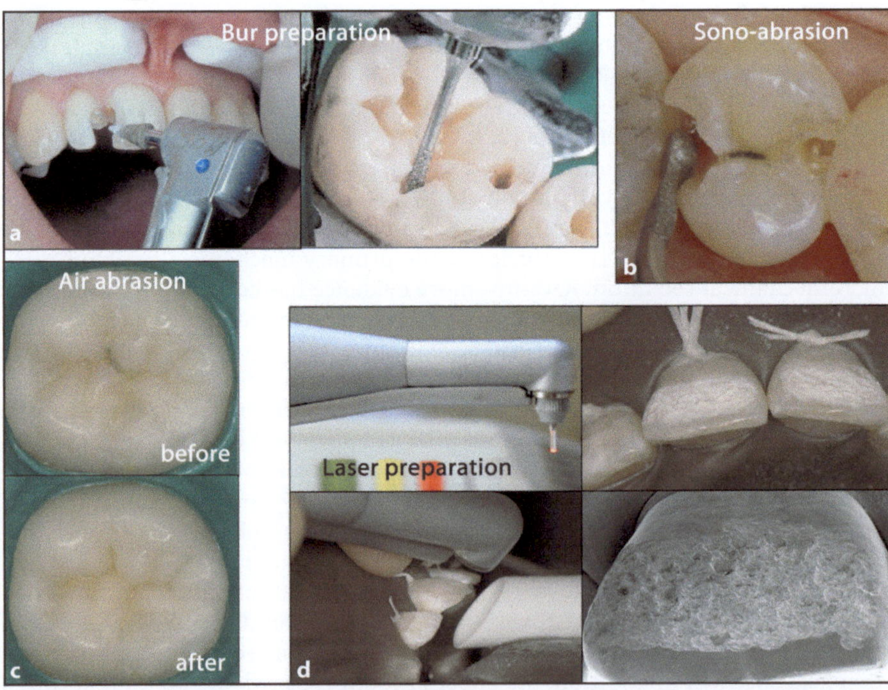

Fig. 5.1 a–d. Adhesive dentistry requires adhesion-receptive tooth surfaces. On the whole, burs remain the standard preparation tools; however, alternatives for dental burs have recently gained attention. Every cavity preparation technique has its own advantages and disadvantages

is difficult, and adjacent teeth are often touched and damaged by the bur [18]. These drawbacks of rotary instruments for cavity preparation, along with the current trend towards "minimal invasiveness" [19–21] have led to the introduction of new tools or the revival of already existing techniques, such as sono-abrasion, air abrasion, and laser ablation (Fig. 5.1) [16, 22].

In the first section, the smear layer in general and its properties are discussed. The following sections deal with various forms of smear layers according to the cavity-preparation technique employed.

Smear Layer

Most commonly, the tooth surface to which the bond will occur is covered with a smear layer. A smear layer is an adherent layer of debris on tooth surfaces when they are cut with rotary or hand instruments [23]. After bur preparation of a cavity, the cavity walls are covered with a smear layer. Endodontic preparation of a root canal, either by rotary or hand instruments, or extensive root planing as periodontal treatment [24], also produce a smear layer in the root canal or on the root surface, respectively. For research purposes, a smear layer is often created in the standard way by grinding the tooth surface with silicon carbide paper.

The smear layer is revealed by scanning electron microscopy (SEM) as a 1- to 2-µm layer of debris with a mainly granular substructure that entirely covers the dentin (Fig. 5.2) [25]. Looking on top of the smear layer, its appearance is generally amorphous, but after sonication, a structure partially composed of aggregates of globular subunits of approximately 0.05–0.1 µm in diameter is exposed [25]. The orifices of the dentin tubules are obstructed by debris tags, called smear plugs, which may extend into the tubule to a depth of 1–10 µm [25, 26]. These smear plugs are contiguous with the smear layer.

The thickness and morphology of the smear layer probably varies with the method used for producing the smear layer and with the location within dentin in relation to the pulp. Tani and Finger [27] have examined light-microscopically smear layers generated by diamond burs with different grain size and by silicon carbide (SiC) papers with varying grit numbers. They concluded that the smear layer's thickness increases with increasing roughness of the diamond bur or SiC paper. A regular grit bur with a grain size of 100 µm (ISO number 806314141504014), often used in clinical cavity preparations, creates a smear layer of 2.2±0.5 µm.

Due to its small and varying dimensions, and irregular and weak structure, studying the smear layer is complicated. The composition of the smear layer has not yet been well defined, but it presumably reflects the composition of the underlying dentin from which it is produced [25]. This was confirmed by Ruse and Smith [28] who used X-ray photo-electron microscopy to examine instrumented dentin. While cutting dentin, the heat and shear forces produced by the rotary movement of the bur cause dentin debris to compact and aggregate. The smear layer is believed to consist of shattered and crushed hydroxyapatite, as well as fragmented and denatured collagen.

In clinical conditions a smear layer may also be contaminated by bacteria and saliva [29–31]. Another disadvantage of a smear layer covering the bonding

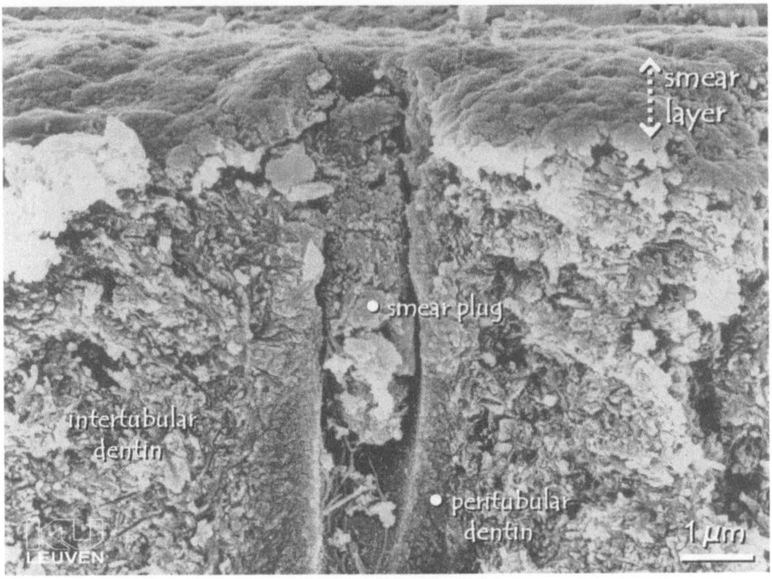

Fig. 5.2. Field-emission scanning electron microscopy photomicrograph a lateral dentin section. The dentin surface has been prepared by wet grinding. A smear layer of approximately 1 μm covers the entire dentin surface, and a smear plug, extending several micrometers into the dentin tubule, occludes the tubule's orifice. The smear layer is an aggregate of mainly fragmented and compacted tooth material and debris. At the surface, the smear layer's appearance is amorphous. (From PhD thesis of J. Perdigão, Katholieke Universiteit, Leuven, 1995)

surface is its inherently weak bond to the underlying dentin [32] and its brittle nature [33]. Early smear-layer incorporating non-acidic adhesives, applied without prior etching, did not penetrate deeply enough to establish a bond with intact dentin. Such bonds were prone to cohesive failure of the smear layer [26, 34].

There are basically two options to overcome low bond strengths due to the limited strength of the smear layer, i.e. removal of the smear layer prior to bonding, or the use of bonding agents that can penetrate beyond the smear layer while incorporating it [35]. Both techniques have been proven successful [36]. Removal of the smear layer, however, increases the permeability of the dentin tubules radically, thereby permitting fluid flow from outside the pulp chamber, and vice versa. Pashley [37] suggested a mainly outward fluid flow under pulpal pressure of 20–70 cm/H_2O. When dentin is covered with an iatrogenically produced smear layer, and the dentin tubules are occluded with smear plugs, fluid permeability is almost reduced to zero [26]. After removal of the smear layer by an acid, dentin permeability through the dentin tubules increases by more than 90% [38–40]. It was feared that removal of the smear layer and subsequent wetting of the dentin surface would affect bond strength between dentin and composite, as the dentinal fluid would dilute primer and bonding agents [41] and as water contamination of bonding was known to lower the bond strength [42]; however, several contemporary systems can cope with augmented fluid permeability of dentin after smear layer removal, and a high and durable bond strength can be achieved [43]. As the

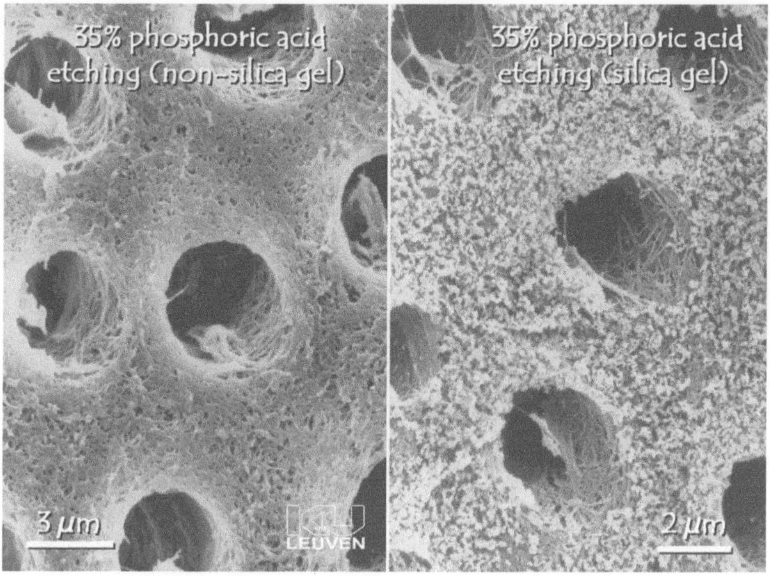

Fig. 5.3. Field-emission scanning electron microscopy photomicrograph of dentin etched with 35% phosphoric acid. Along with removal of the smear layer and smear plugs, the dentin tubules are widened and a porous network of collagen fibrils is exposed. Note the incomplete removal of silica in the right image, despite thorough rinsing. (From PhD thesis of J. Perdigão, Katholieke Universiteit, Leuven, 1995)

main mechanism of tooth sensitivity is based on hydro-dynamic fluid movement, treatment of tooth surfaces to remove the smear layer can induce tooth sensitivity in vivo [33, 44]. It has been suggested that adhesive techniques that require smear-layer removal are associated more with post-operative sensitivity than systems that leave the smear layer in situ [33, 44–46]. Open dentin tubuli may also permit access of bacteria towards the pulp and irritation of the pulp by toxic chemicals such as acids. Although it has been shown that the bonding procedure may cause transient pulpal inflammation, certainly in deep cavities, a continuous bacterial irritation due to microgaps and microleakage is more likely to cause damage to the pulp and post-operative pain [47]. Advantages and disadvantages of removing the smear layer were discussed by Pashley [33]. The first adhesives achieving clinically acceptable results were based on smear layer removal (etch-and-rinse adhesives), but recently new smear-layer incorporating adhesives (self-etch adhesives) have regained popularity [36].

Complete or partial removal of the smear layer can be achieved by applying acidic or chelating solutions called dentin conditioners. In research conditions, sonication has also been used [25]. The more acidic and aggressive the conditioner, the more completely the smear layer and smear plugs will be removed [26, 48]. Strong acids do not only remove the smear layer; they also demineralize intact dentin along with removal of smear plugs to a depth of 1–5 µm, while widening the dentin tubule orifices (Fig. 5.3). Contemporary etch-and-rinse adhesives usually

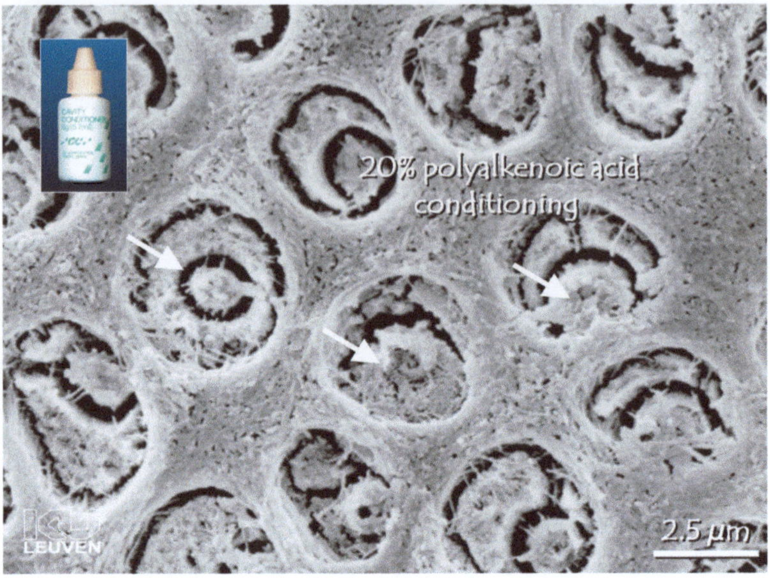

Fig. 5.4. Field-emission scanning electron microscopy photomicrograph of a dentin surface conditioned with 20% polyalkenoic acid. This weak acid has removed the smear layer but has not opened the tubules completely (*arrows*)

use a phosphoric acid gel of 30–40% for the conditioning step. Tested alternatives are maleic acid, nitric acid, citric acid, and tannic acid in varying concentrations. A polyalkenoic acid conditioner used in glass ionomer restorative techniques also provides clean dentin surfaces, although without substantial dentin demineralization [49] and without rendering dentin tubules patent (Fig. 5.4) [50]. Whereas NaOCl is applied to remove organic remnants and bacteria in root canals, chelating agents are widely used in endodontics to remove smear debris produced during the canal preparation. Most commonly, a neutral solution of ethylene diamine tetra-acetic acid is used for removing the smear layer in the root canal [51, 52]. Researchers have been aware for a long time of the presence of a smear layer, and a consensus exists on the fact that the smear layer should be simulated in in vitro research on adhesives. For practical reasons, a smear layer is often prepared by grinding a tooth with a SiC paper. Very often, a SiC paper of 600 grit is applied; however, Tani and Finger [27] demonstrated that the thickness of a smear layer produced by 600-grit SiC is not comparable to that of a smear layer produced with a regular grit bur with a grain size of 100 μm, often used in clinical situations. Sandpapers of 600 sandpapers create thin smear layers (1.2 μm), whereas SiC paper of 180–240 grit is more appropriate to simulate a coarse and clinically relevant smear layer. Koibuchi et al. [53] showed how the use of 600-grit paper could lead to overestimated bond strength when using a self-etch adhesive. Moreover, Tagami indicated a difference in acid resistance between a smear layer produced by bur or by SiC paper grinding [40]. Van Meerbeek et al. [16] demonstrated that dentin surfaces prepared by bur or by wet sanding with SiC paper differ; therefore, it is concluded that a smear layer on dentin intended for in vitro research is best created by a diamond bur.

Sono-Abrasion

Recently, sono-abrasion (SonicSys, Germany, KaVo; PiezzonMaster 400, Switzerland, EMS) has been introduced as an alternative for preparing minimally invasive cavities (Fig. 5.5). This technique is based on the removal of tooth material by an air-driven hand piece equipped with a diamond-coated working tip that removes tooth material by ultrasonic kinetic energy. Different sizes and shapes of diamond tips have been designed, enabling easy access to occlusal and approximal tooth lesions. As these tips are coated only on one side, additional damage and trauma of the approximal side of adjacent teeth is prevented [54, 55].

Considering the semi-rotary movement of the tip, the very high frequency of oscillations of the tip and the subsequently produced heat, dentin exposed by sono-abrasion can also be assumed to be covered by a smear layer (Fig. 5.6). Although few studies have been published, research has pointed out that sono-

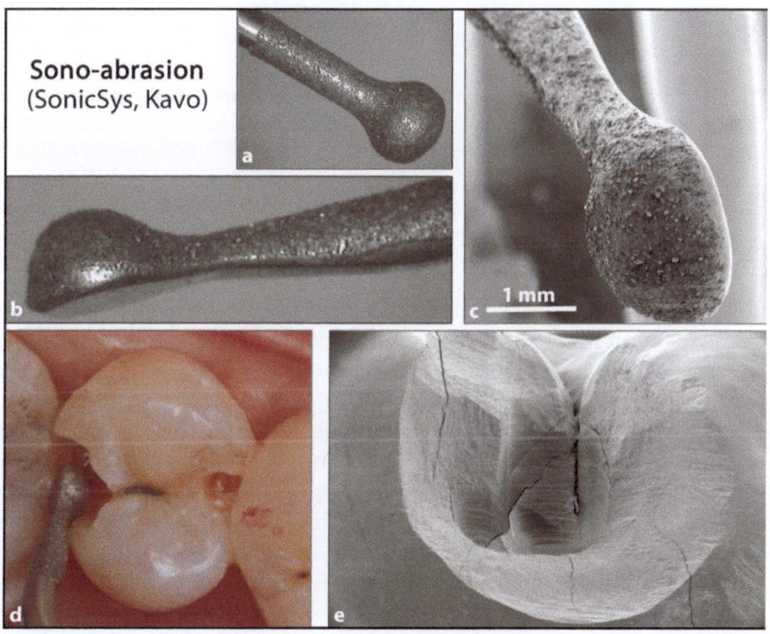

Fig. 5.5. a, b Diamond-coated tip of the SonicSys system (Kavo). Only one side is coated with diamonds, so as to prevent damage to adjacent teeth. The constricted shape of the tip enables easy access in small occlusal and approximal cavities. **c** Field-emission scanning electron microscopy photomicrograph of the same tip. **d** Clinical situation of two class-II cavities. Sono-abrasion can be used for beveling the cavity margins, thereby improving the marginal adaptation of a composite filling. **e** Field-emission scanning electron microscopy photomicrograph of small class-II cavity entirely prepared by sono-abrasion

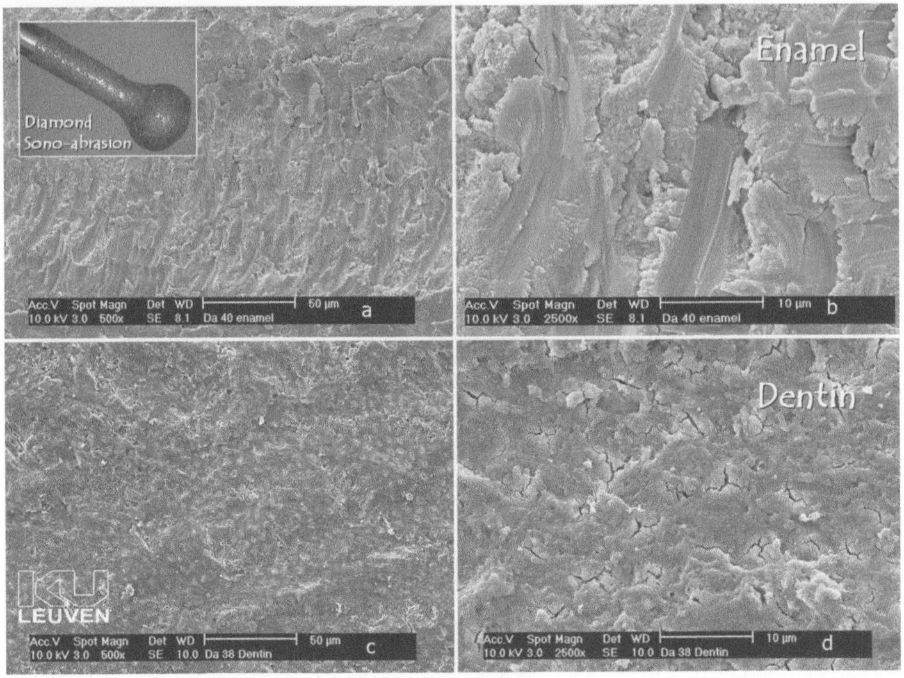

Fig. 5.6 a–d. Field-emission scanning electron microscopy photomicrographs of enamel and dentin surfaces prepared with diamond sono-abrasion. Note the coarse scratches in enamel. Dentin is covered with a relatively thin smear layer and the tubules are occluded by smear plugs

abraded tooth surfaces are indeed very similar to bur-cut dentin. Van Meerbeek et al. [16] found that sono-abrasion resulted in enamel and dentin surfaces equally receptive towards bonding as compared with bur-cut surfaces; however, they also found that a three-step etch-and-rinse adhesive (Optibond FL; Kerr) with omission of the acid-conditioning phase obtains higher bond strengths when bonded to sono-abraded dentin than to bur-cut dentin. This was explained by the relatively high acidity of the primer of Optibond FL (pH=1.78), which thus acts as a self-etch adhesive, and by the fact that sono-abrasion presumably produces rather thin smear layers. Pioch et al. [56] investigated the interface of an etch-and-rinse adhesive with confocal laser scanning microscopy and did not see any difference between bur-prepared or sono-abraded dentin of primary teeth. Opdam et al. [54] reported equal microleakage in class-II cavities prepared by bur or SonicSys, respectively. Their study was confirmed by the findings of Setien [57].

In conclusion, sono-abrasion should be regarded as a good complement to rotary instruments for cavity preparation, the main advantages being less damage to adjacent teeth and minimally invasive cavities. A sono-abraded dentin surface is also covered by a thin smear layer.

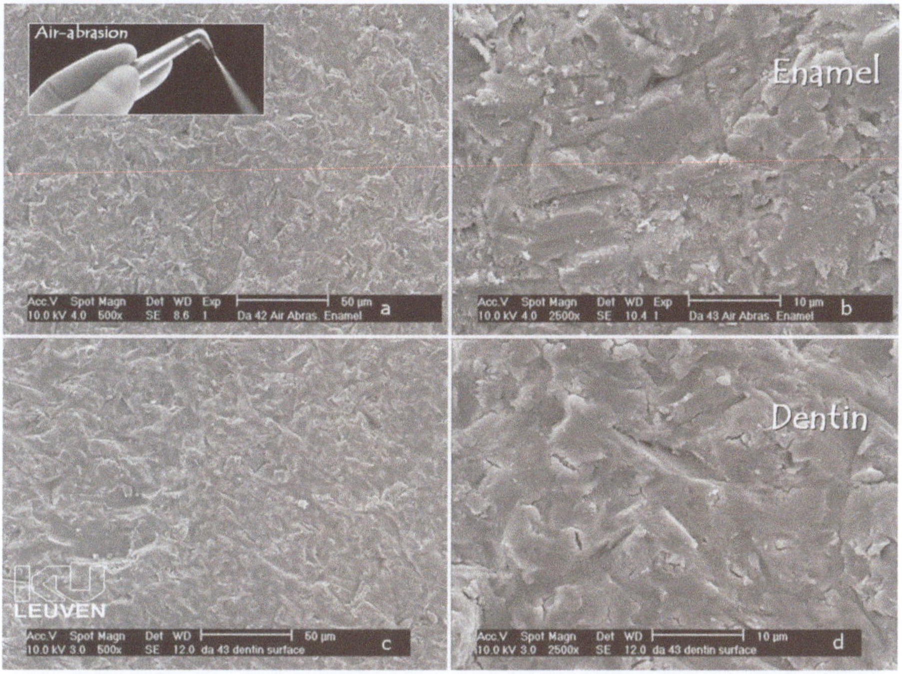

Fig. 5.7 a–d. Field-emission scanning electron microscopy photomicrographs of enamel and dentin prepared by air abrasion. As a result of the kinetic energy of the Al_2O_3 particles fired at the tooth surface, tooth material is chipped away. The resultant enamel (**a**, **b**) and dentin (**c**, **d**) surfaces are very irregular and covered with a discrete smear layer. The dentin tubules are occluded by smear plugs

Air Abrasion

Air abrasion is a relatively old technique that only recently has regained attention. Basically, this technique can be regarded as a small version of sandblasting, which has many applications in common procedure. This technique is already widely used by prosthodontists and dental technicians, for purposes such as increasing surface roughness and enhancing adhesion. Air abrasion is specifically designed for abrading tooth material. The major benefit of this technique is that kinetic energy generated by a high-velocity stream of aluminum oxide particles can be utilized to prepare hard tooth tissues while having little effect on soft materials such as gingival tissues. In addition, this abrasive technique increases patient comfort by reducing heat, vibration, and noise, as commonly experienced during mechanical preparation of teeth when rotating burs are used [16, 58]. The main disadvantages of this technique are in the problems involving removal of the dust particles.

When applied on dentin, air abrasion creates a very irregular surface and a discrete smear layer with smear plugs (Fig 5.7) [16]. Intertubular dentin seems to be impact folded and compressed over the dentin tubules [59]. Although many manufacturers have claimed that an air-abraded tooth surface is more receptive to bonding because of the microretentive surface created by air abrasion, and that the acid-conditioning step can be omitted, many authors have refuted and disproved this [16, 57, 60, 61].

Laser Ablation

Laser technology has gained popularity over the past several years, and many applications in dentistry and medicine have been proposed. One of those applications is caries removal and cavity preparation. Like air abrasion, the trembling experience caused by bur cutting is omitted, rendering this technique more tolerable for patients. In particular, the Erbium:YAG laser with an ultra short square pulse technology (wavelength 2.94 µm) is used as an alternative for cavity preparation, but also Nd:YAG laser can be applied [62, 63].

Laser technology can remove tooth substrate effectively and precisely by means of a thermo-mechanical ablation process involving microexplosions [16]. Water cooling is required to prevent cracking and melting of enamel and dentin, and to prevent thermal damage to the pulp [64].

Laser preparation of tooth substrate does not yield a smear layer [16, 65]. SEM characterization of dentin prepared by Erbium:YAG laser reveals a typical scaly, coarse and irregular surface due to microexplosions and volatilization of tooth material [16, 66–68]. As with air abrasion, laser manufacturers often claim that laser pre-treatment on tooth tissue enhances bonding receptivity of this substrate, and that "laser etching" is able to replace an additional conditioning phase (with phosphoric acid).

Many authors have reported advantages of laser cavity preparation. The acquired rough surface, not demineralized but exhibiting patent dentin tubules, might enhance micromechanical retention [69, 70]. Comparing laser-prepared dentin with bur-cut dentin, similar or better results were found for laser-prepared dentin, regarding bond strength testing [71] and microleakage [70, 72, 73]. Despite these favorable findings concerning laser ablation, increasingly more researchers have changed their opinion regarding the usefulness of lasers for tooth tissue removal. Kataumi et al. [65] were the first to observe substructural cracks in dentin after the use of erbium:YAG laser. Other authors also mention laser damage of enamel and dentin, as more cohesive fractures occur in dentin (Fig. 5.8) [16, 74–76]. Controlled microtensile bond strength tests showed significantly lower bonding effectiveness to lased enamel and dentin [67, 75, 77].

Moreover, this structural weakening is not only confined to the uppermost layer of dentin, but laser irradiation also modifies and weakens dentin over a thickness of 3–5 µm, which understandably jeopardizes adhesion of composite material. In addition, transmission electron microscopy (TEM) investigation of irradiated dentin by Ceballos et al. [67] showed a dense but fissured layer devoid of collagen fibrils. Only in the basal part of this layer were remnants of melted, fused and denatured collagen fibrils found, which were poorly attached to the underlying intact dentin. As interfibrillar spaces were lacking in this zone, resin infiltration must have been impeded, thereby having hindered good adhesion.

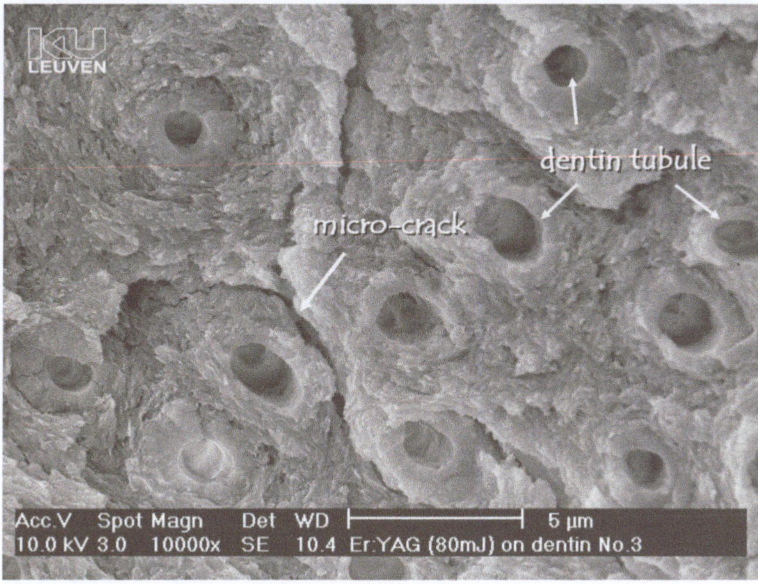

Fig. 5.8. Scanning electron microscopy photomicrograph of laser-conditioned dentin. Laser preparation does not yield a smear layer but gives rise to a microretentive non-demineralized dentin surface with patent tubules; however, adhesion of composites to laser-treated tooth tissue is jeopardized by a structural weakening of the top layer due to microcracks

Mechanical removal of this laser-modified superficial layer or removal by acid etching restores bond strengths [67, 75], but only partially as damage and weakening may go beyond the superficial dentin layer. Microleakage studies also indicate less leakage when lased dentin is acid etched prior to bonding [78, 79].

In summary, current lasers do not yet offer any advantage over conventional rotary instruments for cavity preparation, as they may even affect the bonding substrate adversely. A dentist should understand what structural changes in dentin laser preparation entails and should tackle the aforementioned problems, e.g. by removing the exposed layer as well as possible.

Conclusion

A comprehensive knowledge of the structure of dentin and its altered properties after dentin preparation, according to the used preparation technique, should enable a dentist to understand how to achieve satisfactory bonding to dentin.

Research setups should always be based on the clinical situation, in order to be able to validate in vitro research.

The scope of cavity preparation methods has only recently been widened. Many new techniques need more profound examination, as they can greatly influence the clinical outcome of adhesive techniques.

Even when dealing with dentin of a non-carious lesion and when no cavity preparation is required, a dentist must be aware of the biofilm pellicle covering the tooth lesion. To obtain satisfactory bonding, this lesion should be treated to obtain a clean bonding substrate.

Interfaces and Hybridization

Micromorphological characterization of the interface is paramount to gain insight into the bonding mechanism to tooth tissue. As the adhesive interaction process occurs over a couple of micrometers, electron microscopy is preferred on the grounds of the high resolution that can be achieved (1–2 nm). Mainly two different electron microscopy techniques are used: TEM and SEM. The TEM provides highly informative overview images of both the interaction zone with intact dentin and with the resin layers. The SEM images give us a view of a surface, but special specimen preparation methodologies can also provide SEM images of the interface.

Right from the start, adhesive systems have known a large turnover rate. The big business related to these materials, as well as the continuous search for improved techniques and systems, have urged manufacturers into researching and developing new bonding systems. Whereas original simple bonding agents evolved to multi-step systems, recent development focuses on simplification of the application procedure in order to abate technique sensitivity and reduce manipulation time [80].

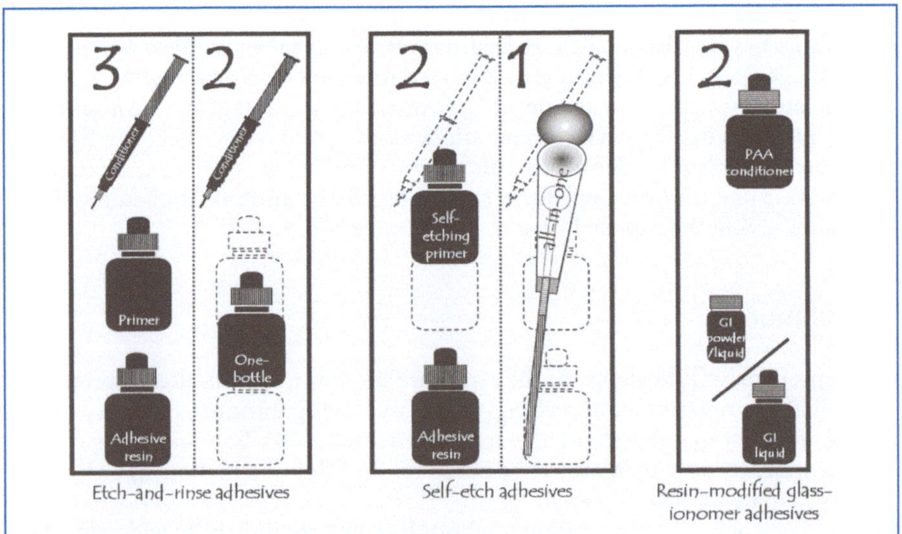

Fig. 5.9. Classification of contemporary adhesives according the adhesion strategy and the clinical application steps

Table 5.1. List of contemporary adhesives categorized following the classification presented in Fig. 5.9

Brand name	Manufacturer
Three-step etch-and-rinse adhesives	
All-Bond 2	Bisco (Schaumburg, Illinois)
Clearfil Liner Bond	Kuraray (Kurashiki, Japan)
Denthesive	Heraeus-Kulzer (Wehrheim, Germany)
EBS	ESPE (now 3 M ESPE; Seefeld, Germany)
Gluma CPS	Bayer (now Heraeus-Kulzer; Leverkusen, Germany)
Optibond DC	Kerr (Orange, Calif.)
Optibond DC	Kerr (Orange, Calif.)
Permagen	Ultradent (Salt Lake City, Utah)
Permaquik	Ultradent
Scotchbond Multi-Purpose	3 M (now 3 M ESPE; St. Paul, Minn.)
Two-step etch-and-rinse adhesives	
C36 Prime&Bond NT	Dentsply-Detrey (Konstanz, Germany)
Excite	Vivadent (Schaan, Lichtenstein)
Gluma 2000	Bayer (now Heraeus-Kulzer; Leverkusen, Germany)
One-Coat Bond	Coltène Whaledent (Altstätten, Switzerland)
One-Step	Bisco (Schaumburg, Illinois)
Optibond Solo Plus	Kerr (Orange, Calif.)
Prime&Bond 2.0	Dentsply-Detrey (Konstanz, Germany)
Prime&Bond 2.1	Dentsply-Detrey (Konstanz, Germany)
Prime&Bond NT	Dentsply-Detrey (Konstanz, Germany)
Scotchbond 1 (Single Bond)	3 M ESPE (Seefeld, Germany)
Solobond M	Voco (Cuxhaven, Germany)
Stae	Southern Dental Industries (Victoria, Australia)
Syntac Single-Component	Ivoclar Vivadent (Schaan, Liechtenstein)
Two step self-etch adhesives	
AdheSE	Ivoclar Vivadent (Schaan, Liechtenstein)
ART Bond	Coltène Whaledent (Altstätten, Switzerland)
Clearfil Liner Bond 2	Kuraray (Osaka, Japan)
Clearfil SE	Kuraray (Osaka, Japan)
Denthesive 2	Heraeus-Kulzer (Wehrheim, Germany)
NRC Prime&Bond NT	Dentsply-Detrey (Konstanz, Germany)
One Coat SE Bond	Coltène Whaledent (Altstätten, Switzerland)
Perme Bond F	Degussa (Hanau, Germany)
Prisma Universal Bond 3	Dentsply-Detrey (Konstanz, Germany)
Pro Bond	Dentsply-Detrey (Konstanz, Germany)
Protect Bond	Kuraray (Osaka, Japan)
Solobond Plus	Voco (Cuxhaven, Germany)
Syntac	Ivoclar Vivadent (Schaan, Liechtenstein)
Tokuso Mac Bond II	MAC (Tokuyama, Japan)
Tyrean	Bisco (Schaumburg, Illinois)
Unifil Bond	GC (Tokyo, Japan)

Table 5.1. (Continued)

Brand name	Manufacturer
One-step self-etch adhesives	
Admira Bond	Voco (Cuxhaven, Germany)
Adper Prompt	3 M ESPE (Seefeld, Germany)
AQ Bond	Sun Medical (Shiga, Japan)
Etch&Prime 3.0	Degussa (Hanau, Germany)
Sustel/ F2000 primer-adhesive	3 M ESPE (Seefeld, Germany)
Futurabond	Voco (Cuxhaven, Germany)
Hytac OSB	ESPE (Seefeld, Germany)
iBond	Heraeus-Kulzer (Wehrheim, Germany)
One-Up Bond F	Tokuyama (Tokyo, Japan)
Prime&Bond 2.1 (without etching)	Dentsply-Detrey (Konstanz, Germany)
Prime&Bond NT (without etching)	Dentsply-Detrey (Konstanz, Germany)
Prompt-L-Pop	3 M ESPE (Seefeld, Germany)
Prompt-L-Pop (LP2)	3 M ESPE (Seefeld, Germany)
PSA	Dentsply-Detrey (Konstanz, Germany)
Reactmer Bond	Shofu (Kyoto, Japan)
Xeno III	Dentsply-Detrey (Konstanz, Germany)
Glass-ionomers	
Exp. Vitremer (Primer)	3 M ESPE (Seefeld, Germany)
Fuji Cap II	GC (Tokyo, Japan)
Fuji 2 LC (GC Dentin conditioner)	GC (Tokyo, Japan)
Fuji Bond LC (GC Cavity conditioner)	GC (Tokyo, Japan)
Fuji Bond LL	GC (Tokyo, Japan)
HIFI Master Palette (HI Tooth cleanser)	Shofu (Kyoto, Japan)
Ketac-fil (Ketac conditioner)	ESPE (now 3 M ESPE; Seefeld, Germany)
Photac-fil (Ketac conditioner)	ESPE (now 3 M ESPE; Seefeld, Germany)
Vitremer (Vitremer Primer)	3 M ESPE (Munich, Germany)

Classifying dental adhesives in different categories is not straightforward, because of the great supply and vast turnover of adhesives. Several classifications have been suggested in the past in scientific literature; however, no consensus concerning terminology has been reached yet. Van Meerbeek et al. [4, 36] have suggested a scientifically based classification with three main groups of adhesives: etch-and-rinse adhesives, self-etch adhesives and glass-ionomer adhesives (Fig. 5.9; Table 1). This classification is simple and has proved to be reliable and consistent. As it is based on the applied adhesion strategy, this classification provides a dentist or a researcher with background information on the adhesion mechanism and on the characteristics of an adhesive system; therefore, from this point forward, we discuss adhesives and their interaction with dentin, grouped according to the three main divisions of this classification.

All three categories of adhesives exhibit a common adhesion mechanism of hybridization. This is the process of micromechanical interlocking ensuring a demineralization, infiltration and polymer setting process, and was first described by Nakabayashi et al. [81]. A hybrid layer is the resulting resin-infiltrated surface layer of dentin (and enamel).

Etch-and-Rinse Adhesives

Etch-and-rinse adhesives can readily be recognized by an initial etching step, the so-called conditioning step, followed by a compulsory rinsing phase. Another frequently used name for this category of adhesives is "total-etch" adhesives [80, 82], which is, however, less appropriate because self-etch adhesives can also etch and demineralize tooth tissue.

This etching step demineralizes dentin in order to remove the smear layer and smear plugs, and to achieve a microporous surface with enhanced bonding capacity. To demineralize dentin, both chelating acids and mineral acids can be used [45]. Many different conditioners with varying concentrations have been investigated, such as citric, maleic, nitric, oxalic and phosphoric acid [80]. As etch-and-rinse systems are applied on both enamel and dentin, the etching effectiveness of weak acids or low concentrations on enamel are doubtful. Current etch-and-rinse systems usually use 30–40% phosphoric acid.

Originally, etch-and-rinse systems typically consisted of three separate application steps: (a) conditioning; (b) priming; and (c) adhesive resin application. An adhesive system that follows this procedure is called a three-step etch-and-rinse adhesive. In searching for fewer application steps and simplification, a two-step etch-and-rinse design has been devised (Fig. 5.9) combining the priming and bonding steps into one. Another frequently used name for a two-step etch-and-rinse adhesive is "one-bottle adhesive", misleadingly suggesting a single application step.

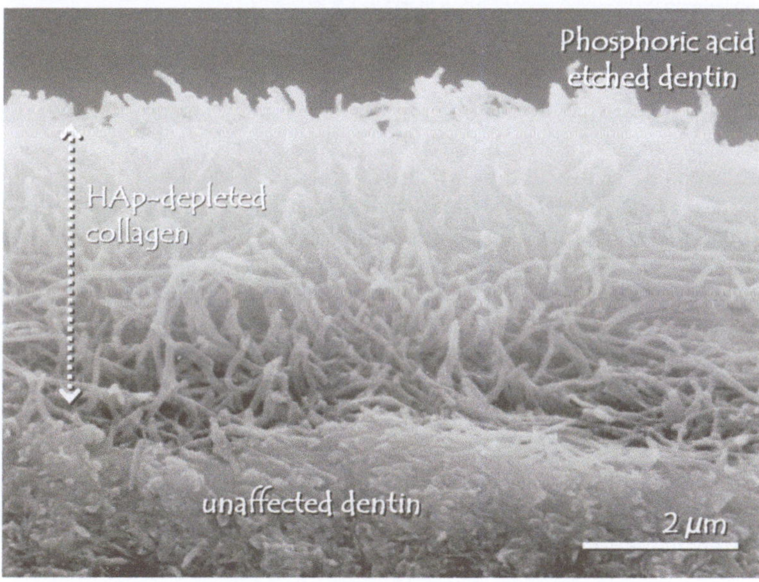

Fig. 5.10. Field-emission scanning electron microscopy photomicrograph of demineralized dentin. Treatment with 35% phosphoric acid for 15 s demineralizes dentin over a depth of 3–5 µm, thereby exposing a scaffold of collagen fibrils that is nearly totally depleted of hydroxyapatite. As a consequence, a retentive network with interfibrillar spaces of approximately 20 nm is created. (Courtesy of M. Vargas, University of Iowa)

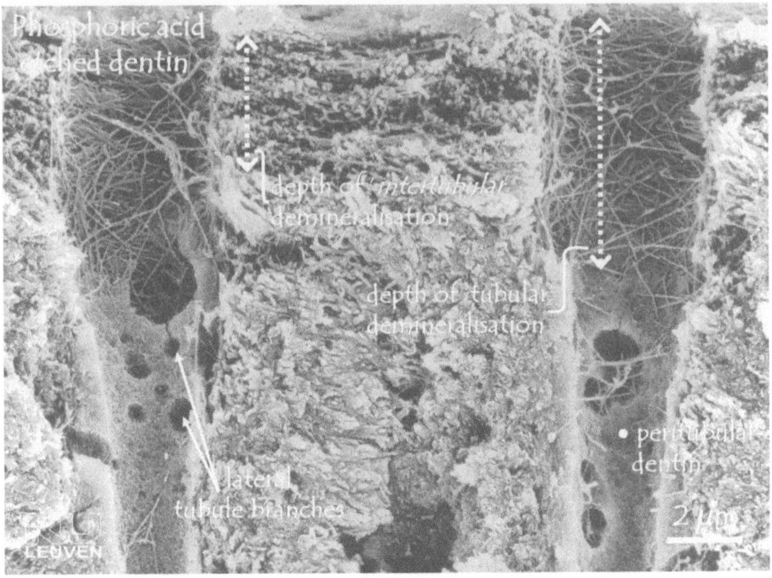

Fig. 5.11. Field-emission scanning electron microscopy image of a cross-section through dentin etched with 37.5% phosphoric acid. At the dentin tubule walls, peritubular dentin has been completely dissolved, resulting in the typical funneling of the tubule orifice. Note that the depth of demineralization in the dentin tubule (6–7 µm) exceeds the depth of intertubular demineralization (3–5 µm). Several orifices of lateral tubule branches can be observed. (From PhD thesis of J. Perdigão, Katholieke Universiteit, Leuven, 1995)

Both three- and two-step etch-and-rinse adhesives pursue a similar adhesion mechanism. In the conditioning step, phosphoric acid removes the smear layer while concurrently demineralizing dentin over a depth of 3–5 µm, thereby exposing a scaffold of collagen fibrils that is nearly totally depleted of hydroxyapatite (Fig. 5.10) [83–86]. As the highly mineralized peritubular dentin is almost completely dissolved, dentin tubules are widened and their orifices become funnel shaped (Fig. 5.11). The exposed collagen fibrils function as a microretentive network for micromechanical interlocking of the resulting resin polymers. When drying acid-etched dentin, this collagen network collapses and shrinks, thereby jeopardizing monomer infiltration [23, 87, 88].

After the conditioning step, adhesion-promoting monomers are applied in one or two application steps to penetrate the exposed collagen network.

The priming step in three-step etch-and-rinse adhesives should ensure sufficient wetting of the exposed collagen fibrils and remove remaining water, thereby preparing dentin for adhesive resin infiltration. A primer solution is a mixture of specific monomers with hydrophilic properties dissolved in organic solvents. HEMA is an important monomer that is very frequently added to these primer solutions. Due to its low molecular weight and hydrophilic nature, HEMA promotes resin infiltration into and re-expansion of the collagen network [89], thereby improving bond strength of the adhesive [90].

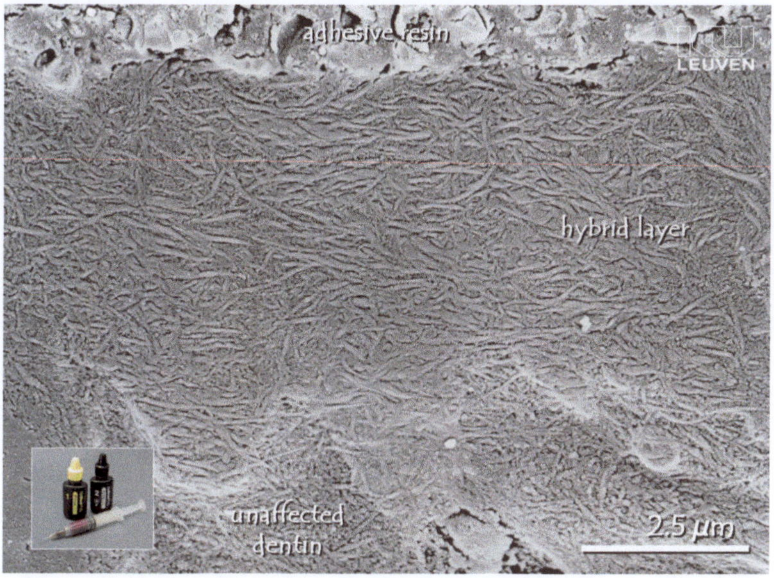

Fig. 5.12. Field-emission scanning electron microscopy photomicrograph of a diamond-knife-sectioned resin–dentin interface produced by the three-step etch-and-rinse adhesive Optibond FL (Kerr). The loosely arranged collagen fibrils in the 3- to 5-µm-thick hybrid layer are easily recognizable

The adhesive resin is a solvent-free, filled or unfilled (i.e. containing filler particles) solution containing mainly hydrophobic monomers. The main function of this adhesive resin is to fill up the interfibrillar spaces left between the collagen fibrils. Upon curing and polymerization of these monomers, a hybrid layer and resin tags are created that provide micromechanical retention (Figs. 5.12–5.14) [91]. In two-step self-etch adhesives, priming and adhesive bonding components are combined into one solution that should fulfill both functions.

Neither the thickness of the hybrid layer nor the length of the resin tags seems to play an important role regarding the bond strength [7, 92]. True chemical adhesion between collagen and the methacrylate monomers is unlikely, because of the inert nature of collagen fibrils and the low affinity of the monomers for hydroxyapatite-depleted collagen [80].

Thus far, in vitro and in vivo research has pointed out that etch-and-rinse adhesives can achieve high-quality adhesion to both enamel and dentin [93]. In in vitro and in clinical studies, three-step etch-and-rinse adhesives perform superiorly to two-step etch-and-rinse adhesives [92, 94, 95]; the latter are also associated with greater technique sensitivity than their three-step counterparts, which is understandable as a single solution combines the two separate functions of primer and bonding resin [96]. Moreover, after aging procedures in durability studies, the bonding integrity of three-step etch-and-rinse adhesives is better

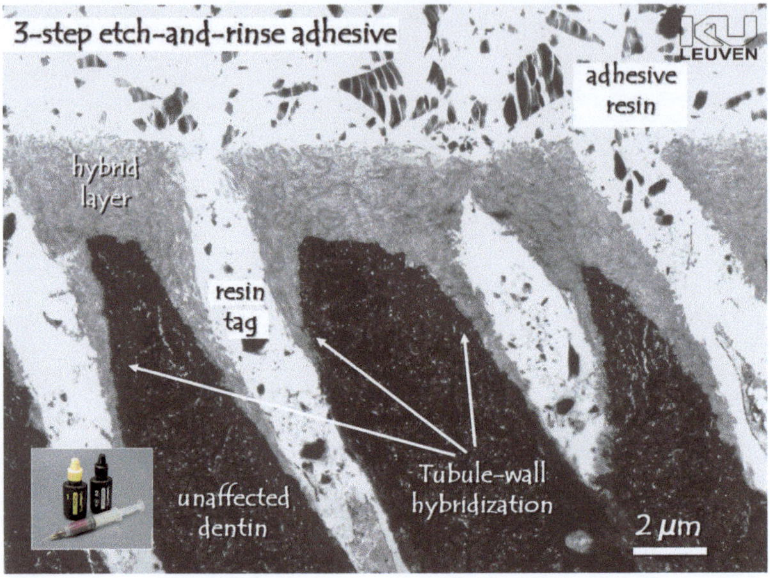

Fig. 5.13. Transmission electron microscopy photomicrograph of the interface produced by Optibond (Kerr). Note that the hybrid layer extends into the dentinal tubules, attaching the resin tags to the tubules walls. "Tubule-wall hybridization" is considered important for the hermetic sealing of the pulp against microleakage

maintained [43]; therefore, three-step etch-and-rinse adhesives are often considered as the standard among adhesives. As two-step etch-and-rinse adhesives do not really involve a time-saving or improved performance, their use does not hold advantages and should be discouraged.

Technique sensitivity of etch-and-rinse systems in general is their major drawback. Most difficulties are related to the etch-and-rinse phase. Firstly, technique sensitivity can in part be attributed to the susceptibility of the collagen scaffold to collapse, thus impeding proper infiltration of the collagen with monomers [87, 97, 98]. Etching dentin removes the mineral phase completely, leaving the collagen fibrils suspended in water. Whereas enamel should preferentially be dry to achieve good bonding, a certain amount of water is needed to prevent the collagen fibrils in dentin from shrinking (Fig. 5.15). To overcome this problem and to maintain the structural integrity of interfibrillar spaces in the collagen network, two different approaches can be followed, depending on the primer of the adhesive system [4, 99].

The first approach, known as "dry-bonding" technique, involves air drying of dentin after acid etching, and applying a water-based primer, capable of re-expanding the collapsed collagen meshwork [100, 101]. An alternative approach is to leave dentin moist, thereby preventing any collapse and using an acetone-based primer, known for its water-chasing capacity. This technique is commonly referred to as "wet bonding" and was introduced by Kanca, and by Gwinnett et al., in the 1990s [102–104]; however, determining how moist the dentin should be to

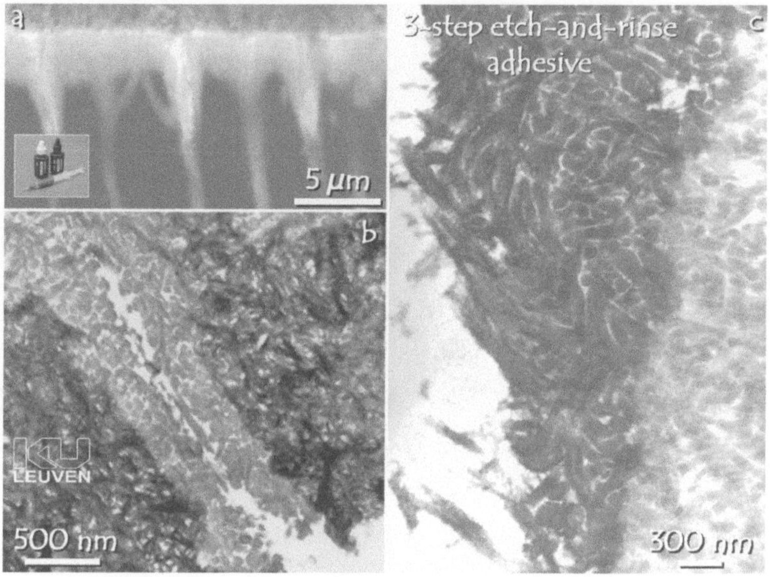

Fig. 5.14. **a** Laser scanning confocal photomicrograph illustrates the resin–dentin interface of Optibond (Kerr). The adhesive resin component of Optibond is labeled with rhodamine B. Note the formation of microresin tags in the lateral tubular branches. **b** Detail of transmission electron microscopy photomicrograph of a non-demineralized dentin section, showing a microresin tag. A narrow core of resin is surrounded by a hybridized wall ("lateral tubule hybridization"). **c** Transmission electron microscopy photomicrograph of a demineralized and stained dentin section, showing a close-up of the thin hybrid layer produced in the wall of dentin tubules ("tubule-wall hybridization"). Note the typical cross-banding of the collagen fibrils and their fraying ends, called "shag-carpet" appearance

ensure complete water removal by the acetone-based primer is complicated. Problems resulting from excess of water have been described by Tay [105, 106] and have been coined "overwetting phenomena" [107]. Because the "dry-bonding" technique is significantly less sensitive to variations in application procedure [101] and does not compromise bonding effectiveness [100], it should be preferred over the hard-to-standardize wet-bonding technique.

Even when preventing collapse, or when re-expanding after drying, incomplete resin infiltration of the hydroxyapatite-depleted collagen can occur [10]. Especially over etching with subsequent deep demineralization can lead to suboptimal resin impregnation and to a porous zone in the hybrid layer [10, 108]. In the long run, this may compromise the durability of the bond [109–111]. The nanoleakage phenomenon (Fig. 16), which is basically the presence of submicrometer-sized gaps within the hybrid layer [98] that are disclosed by interface staining with silver tracers, is considered as a manifestation of incomplete resin infiltration of the hybrid layer and of a discrepancy between the depth of demineralization and the depth of resin infiltration. An alternative explanation for nanoleakage in the hybrid layer is the poor adaptation and envelopment of the resin to the collagen fibrils, leaving microscopic gaps [36].

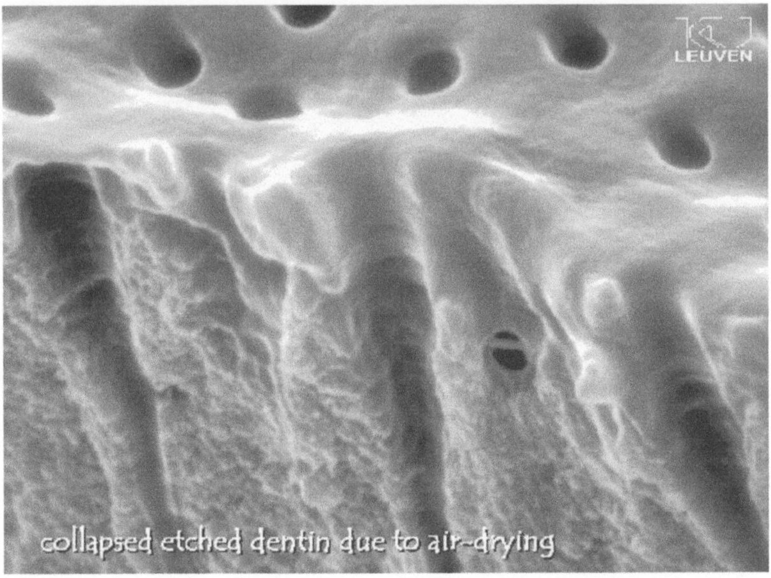

Fig. 5.15. Lateral view of phosphoric-acid-etched dentin by FL. SEM. The exposed collagen network is susceptible to shrinkage and has collapsed due to air drying. Note that no interfibrillar spaces are left and that subsequent resin infiltration will be hindered

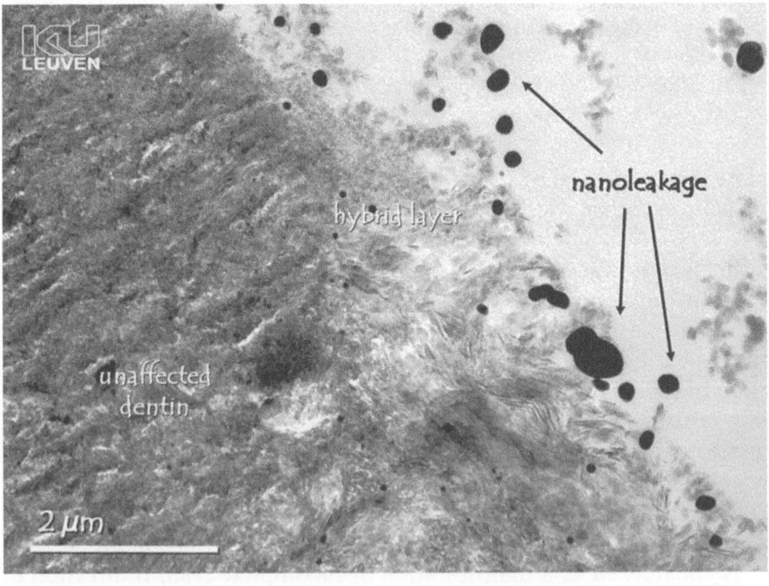

Fig. 5.16. Example of nanoleakage. Transmission electron microscopy photomicrograph of a non-demineralized dentin section stained with silver nitrate. Due to its low molecular weight, silver nitrate is capable of penetrating into very small discrepancies. Such silver tracers are therefore used to search for submicron gaps within the hybrid layer

This class of adhesives is also sensitive to humidity and contamination, making the use of cofferdam in clinical patient treatment indispensable [112]. In particular, HEMA-containing adhesives have been reported to be influenced by water [42].

In summary, three-step etch-and-rinse adhesives are considered as the gold standard, and despite the elaborate and lengthy working procedure, and the technique sensitivity associated with acetone-based adhesives, they can achieve very satisfactory results. Dentists should, however, be aware of their weak points, and adapt their application procedure accordingly.

Self-Etch Adhesives

Although the self-etch concept is not new [4], it has only recently come under extensive scrutiny. First self-etch adhesives were developed by raising the amount of acidic monomers in HEMA-water based adhesives [82]. Self-etch adhesives do not require a separate "etch-and-rinse" phase, as they contain acidic monomers that simultaneously condition and prime enamel and dentin. As a result, the dissolved smear layer and demineralization products are not rinsed away but incorporated in the adhesive resin [113, 114].

Self-etch adhesives can be subdivided according to their application procedure (see Fig. 5.9) and their acidity and aggressiveness [4, 115]. Similarly to etch-and-rinse adhesives, a two-step and a simplified one-step version of self-etch adhesives exist. Initial self-etch systems consisted of an acidic primer, followed by an adhesive resin. Recently, "all-in-one" adhesives or one-step self-etch adhesives have been brought onto the market which combine etching, priming and conditioning into one solution [116, 117].

The morphological features of the hybrid layer produced by self-etch adhesives depend a great deal on the aggressiveness of the functional monomers [36, 118]. Consequently, three categories of self-etch adhesives can be made according their acidity: mild ($pH \geq 2$); intermediate ($pH \approx 1.5$); and strong self-etch adhesives ($pH \leq 1$; Fig. 5.17) [115, 119, 120]. Mild self-etch adhesives demineralize dentin only very shallowly, leaving hydroxyapatite crystals around the collagen fibrils available for possible chemical interaction. Usually, the smear plug is not completely removed from the dentine tubule. As a result, a shallow hybrid layer is formed with submicron measures (Fig. 5.18). The TEM images of strong self-etch adhesives applied on dentin strongly resemble the morphological aspect of an etch-and-rinse adhesive, with a thick hybrid layer, which is completely devoid of hydroxyapatite crystals, and with resin tags (Fig. 5.19). The more aggressive the adhesive, the deeper hybridization [45]. "Intermediary strong" self-etch adhesives exhibit morphological features that lie between the mild and strong self-etch adhesives. Figure 5.20 demonstrates the interaction of a mild and a strong self-etch primer with smear-layer-covered dentin. Current self-etch adhesives have been proven acidic enough to penetrate beyond the smear layer, even without agitation and within a clinically relevant time [27]; however, apart from the pH of the priming solution, other factors, such as agitation during application, thickness of the smear layer, viscosity and wetting characteristics, also account for the obtained depth of infiltration and demineralization by self-etch adhesives [108, 121].

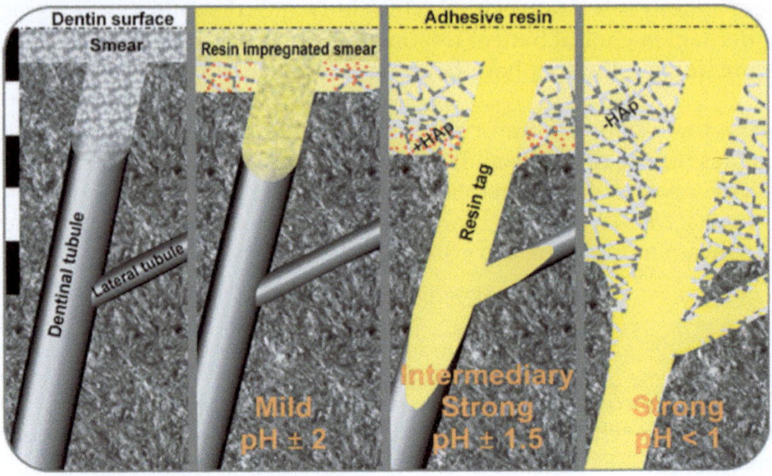

Fig. 5.17. Schematic overview of the interaction of different self-etch adhesives with dentin (*bar at left* represents approximately 5 µm). On the left, unaffected dentin is represented that is covered by a smear layer. On the right, interaction of three classes of self-etch adhesives with dentin and the smear layer is represented. As "mild" self-etch adhesives do not completely remove the smear layer, a relatively thin sub-micron hybrid layer is formed without resin tags. The "intermediary strong" self-etch adhesives remove the smear layer along with a shallow demineralization of dentin. Short resin tags (±10 µm) are formed, and a limited lateral-wall hybridization takes place. In the bottom third of the hybrid layer, not all hydroxyapatite crystals have been dissolved. The micromorphological aspect of "strong" self-etch adhesives is very similar to that of etch-and-rinse adhesives and is characterized by a 3- to 5-µm-thick hybrid layer, dentinal tubules' funneling, extensive resin tags, as well as tubule-wall and lateral tubule-wall hybridization

Despite the small hybrid layer and the absence of resin tags (little micromechanical retention), mild self-etch adhesives can reach satisfactory results as far as bond strength is concerned [36, 92]. Together with the finding that the thickness of the hybrid layer and the presence of resin tags do not overly influence the bonding performance [7, 92], chemical interaction between the monomers and hydroxyapatite may be a plausible explanation for the good performance of self-etch adhesives [5]. The carboxylic and phosphate groups that render these monomers hydrophilic and that function as proton donors, have been proven to bond ionically with calcium in hydroxyapatite [122]. The ability to make chemical bonds is monomer specific and depends on the hydrolytic stability of the calcium-monomer bond. Yoshida et al. have shown using XPS (X-ray photo-electron microscopy) that 10-MDP exceeds the bonding potential of 4-MET and phenyl-P [5]. The hydrolytic stability of the monomer itself is also important, especially with regard to bond durability. Whereas micromechanical retention is thought to provide resistance to "acute" de-bonding stresses, the relevance of additional chemical bonding is suggested to lie in durability and survival of adhesion [4, 36].

The composition of self-etch adhesives is quite unique as they contain high concentrations of water and acidic monomers [118]. Water is an indispensable

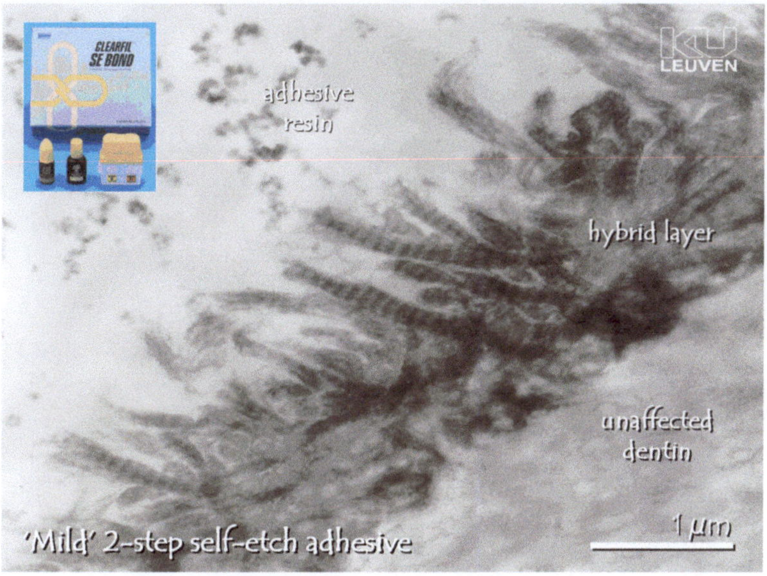

Fig. 5.18. Transmission electron microscopy photomicrograph of a demineralized and stained section through the resin–dentin interface produced by Clearfil SE (Kuraray). Note the formation of a 1-µm-thick hybrid layer and the typical shag-carpet appearance of individual collagen fibrils; these are easily recognizable thanks to their cross-banded appearance

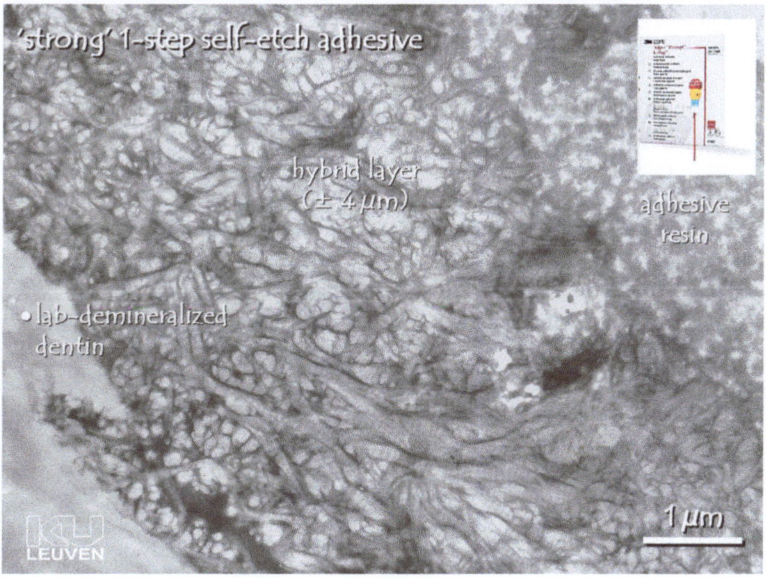

Fig. 5.19. Transmission electron microscopy photomicrograph of a stained demineralized section through the resin–dentin interface produced by the strong one-step self-etch adhesive Adper Prompt (3 M ESPE). Dentin has been relatively deeply demineralized, and no hydroxyapatite crystals remained in the hybrid layer. The demineralization front has stopped abruptly. This image resembles greatly the morphological aspect of an etch-and-rinse adhesive

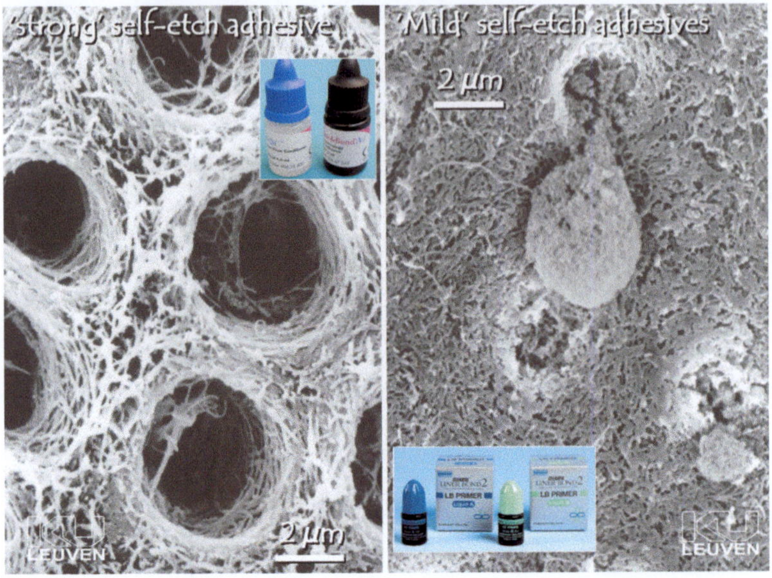

Fig. 5.20. Field-emission scanning electron microscopy image shows the interactions of a "strong" (*left*) and a "mild" (*right*) self-etch primer. The strong self-etch primer (Non-Rinse Conditioner) of Prime&Bond NT (Denstply/Detrey) has removed the smear layer and smear plugs while exposing the collagen network and widening of the tubules' orifices. Conversely, the interaction of the mild self-etch primer of Clearfil Liner Bond 2 (Kuraray) is clearly less intense, as only little collagen is exposed and most of the tubules remain occluded with smear

ingredient of current self-etch systems that provides in an ionization medium for the functional monomers [123]. Two-step self-etch adhesives consist of a hydrophilic aqueous primer solution and a separate hydrophobic adhesive resin. Similar to the combined primer/adhesive resin solution of two-step etch-and-rinse adhesives, one-step self-etch adhesives are complex mixtures of both hydrophilic and hydrophobic components. In particular, the high concentrations of water have raised questions about potentially harmful effects on polymerization, given that incomplete water removal is realistic [42, 123]. This also applies for the high concentrations of solvent that may cause incomplete resin polymerization in case of incomplete evaporation.

While bonding to enamel remains a problem, especially for mild self-etch adhesives [95, 108], bonding to dentin has yielded reasonable results. Some two-step self-etch adhesives have been documented with adequate in vitro bonding strengths that come in the vicinity of that of etch-and-rinse adhesives [92]. Recent studies have also reported good clinical results for some self-etch adhesives. Clearfil SE (Kuraray, Osaka, Japan), which is a mild two-step self-etch adhesive, was reported to have high retention rates in non-carious class-V cavities after 2 years [124, 125] and after 3 years [126].

The great variability between the performance of different self-etch adhesives can in part be ascribed to the use of different functional monomers with different properties, regarding acidity, hydrolytic stability and chemical bonding capacity.

Compared with etch-and-rinse adhesives, many advantages have been appointed to self-etch adhesives. It has been suggested that they improve the efficiency in clinical procedures by omitting the obligatory rinsing phase in etch-and-rinse adhesives, thus reducing the chair-side time [127]. Conditioning, rinsing and drying steps, which may be critical and difficult to standardize in clinical conditions, are eliminated in self-etch adhesives [108]. Technique sensitivity associated with bonding to dehydrated demineralized dentin is eliminated, as a rinsing and drying phase are no longer needed [128]. Collapse of the collagen network is prevented, as monomers infiltrate concomitantly as they demineralize [114, 129, 130]. Another advantage of the attendant demineralization and resin infiltration is that theoretically incomplete resin infiltration is prevented [114, 118]; however, recent nanoleakage observations in the hybrid layer, and especially beyond the hybrid layer, have shed doubt on the concept that self-etch adhesives ensure complete resin infiltration [131]. As the smear layer and smear plugs are not removed prior to the actual bonding procedure, rewetting of dentin by dentinal fluid from the dentin tubules is prevented [132] and potential postoperative sensitivity has been reported to be reduced [123, 125]. Perdigão et al. [133], however, did not observe any difference in postoperative sensitivity between a three-step etch-and-rinse adhesive and a self-etch system. In case of mild self-etch adhesives, which are characterized by a superficial and partial demineralization of dentin, hydroxyapatite crystals are left available in the hybrid layer for possible chemical bonding (Fig. 5.18) [36].

One-step self-etch adhesives (1-SEAs) are undoubtedly the most user-friendly adhesives on market, but they have also been associated with considerable shortcomings. The relatively low bond strengths obtained by 1-SEAs are a main concern. Compared with multi-step self-etch and etch-and-rinse versions, one-step self-etch adhesives consistently achieve lower bond strengths [92, 95, 134, 135]. Due to their high hydrophilicity, cured one-step self-etch adhesives have been demonstrated to act as permeable membranes, permitting water movement across the adhesive layer [136, 137]. Reticular patterns of nanoleakage, so-called water trees, can be found within the adhesive layer of 1-SEAs and are considered as sites of incomplete water removal and subsequent suboptimal polymerized resins [138]. The relevance of these water trees remains unclear, but as they may function as water ducts, they may contribute to accelerated degradation of tooth–resin bonds [138–141]. More recently, complex processes of phase separation have been shown to occur in one-component, HEMA-free SEAs [142]. Adhesive solutions were examined using light microscopy. As soon as the adhesive was dispensed onto a glass plate and solvent started to evaporate, a phase separation occurred, yielding a multitude of droplets that slowly emerged towards the upper surface of the adhesive drop, to finally disappear. If the adhesive was light cured, all remaining droplets were entrapped in the adhesive layer.

The explanation for these observations is in the complex mixture of both hydrophobic and hydrophilic components, dissolved in an organic solvent (usually ethanol or acetone). Gradual evaporation of solvent sets off the phase-separation reaction, in which presumably water separates from the other adhesive ingredients. HEMA plays a key role in this process, as this monomer acts as a wetting agent due to its hydrophilic character and can prevent water from separating from other adhesive ingredients. It is self-evident that incorporation of droplets may contribute to bond degradation, but persistence of water in the adhesive layer may also affect bond strength adversely.

Glass-Ionomer Approach

A third adhesive approach is based on the technology of glass ionomers and their auto-adhesive capacity. Glass ionomers are the only true self-adhesive materials as they can adhere to both enamel and dentin by a specific glass-ionomer interaction. Diverse formulas of glass ionomers are on the market varying in use: glass-ionomer restorative materials, cements and adhesives. Whereas glass-ionomer cements provide adhesion for indirect restorations, glass-ionomer adhesives can be used to bond direct composite restorations.

Glass ionomers have a specific composition, containing polyacrylic acid, alkenoic copolymers, glass-filler particles and water. When resin components are added to glass ionomers, these are called resin-modified glass ionomers. The adhesion reaction to tooth tissue is based mainly on the glass-ionomer components and involves both a micromechanical hybridization and a chemical reaction. In the particular case of glass-ionomer adhesives, which are actually resin-modified glass ionomers, the resin components ensure good bonding with the lining composite.

Regarding bonding mechanism, they can be considered a special group of self-etch adhesives based on glass-ionomer technology. Like self-etch adhesives, their adhesive capacity is twofold and depends both on a limited demineralization of enamel and dentin with subsequent infiltration and mechanical interlocking, and on a chemical adhesion between calcium in hydroxyapatite and polyalkenoic acid [122, 143, 144]. The demineralization reaction is set off by the high molecular weight polyalkenoic acid. This acidic molecule exposes a microporous collagen network by selectively dissolving hydroxyapatite crystals. Additionally, an ionic bonding takes place between the carboxyl groups of the polyalkenoic acid and the calcium of remaining hydroxyapatite crystals. This bond has been proven to be relatively stable, capable of withstanding ultrasonic rinsing [122].

Micromorphologically, a shallow hybrid layer of 0.5–1 µm in thickness is formed (Fig. 5.21). Because of a mild and partial demineralization, hydroxyapatite crystals can be distinguished on the collagen fibrils within the hybrid layer. Typically, a "gel phase" closely attached to the hybrid layer is observed in some glass ionomers. This amorphous phase on top of the interface has been reported to represent salt of calcium polycarboxylate [145].

A conditioning step with a weak polyalkenoic acid (PAA) significantly improves the bond strength [50]. Its beneficial effect on bond strength lies in a threefold mechanism: (a) the removal of the smear layer by PAA; (b) a shallow demineralization of the tooth tissue; and (c) a chemical interaction of PAA with residual hydroxyapatite [122].

Clinically, the good adhesion of glass ionomers and resin-modified glass ionomers is striking. Very high retention rates of more than 90% have been observed for periods up to 5 years in non-carious cervical lesions [94, 126, 146, 147]. Moreover, a recent study has revealed that glass-ionomer retention rates exceed by far the retention rates of other adhesives [126, 148]. Other advantages of glass

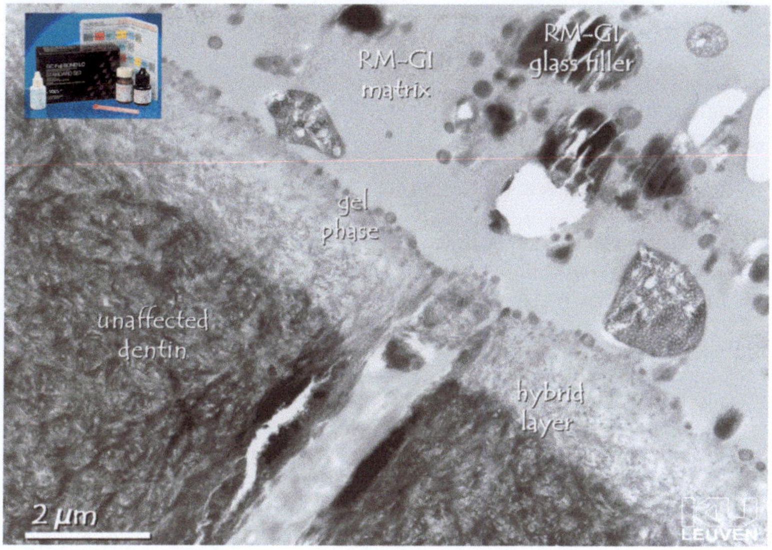

Fig. 5.21. Transmission electron microscopy photomicrograph of an unstained, non-demineralized dentin section, showing the interaction of dentin with Fuji Bond LC (GC). A partially demineralized hybrid layer of approximately 1 µm is formed. The remaining hydroxyapatite crystals within the hybrid layer function as receptors for chemical bonding with the carboxyl groups of the polyalkenoic acid. On top of the hybrid layer, an amorphous, gray "gel phase" represents the reaction product formed through interaction of the polyalkenoic acid with calcium that was extracted from the dentin surface

ionomers are their biocompatibility and their fluoride release. The main drawback of glass-ionomer restorations is their inferior esthetic quality as compared with composites. This disadvantage can, however, be avoided by using a glass-ionomer adhesive and a composite restoration.

Conclusion

A good classification of adhesives is indispensable to keep an overview of the current adhesives. The strength of the proposed classification lies in its simplicity and its scientific basis. Each category in this classification is characterized by a specific bonding mechanism, a specific and distinct application protocol and by a specific ultra-morphological image; however, as for bonding effectiveness, it becomes increasingly clear that an adhesive's in vitro and in vivo performances also greatly depend on its specific ingredient composition.

Despite enhanced ease and faster application, simplified adhesives thus far seem to induce a loss of bonding effectiveness, and their advantages should be weighed off against their shortcomings.

Ultimatelly, the only true criterion for an adhesive's quality is its long-term clinical performance.

Acknowledgements. Kirsten Van Landuyt is appointed as 'Aspirant FWO'. Moreover, some reference to Leuven Biomat Research Cluster (Katholieke University Leuven) should be made as all authors are part of it.

References

1. Summit J, Robbins J, Schwartz R. Operative dentistry: a contemporary approach. Quintessence, Chicago, 2001, p 17
2. Gaengler P, Hoyer I, Montag R, Gaebler P. Micromorphological evaluation of posterior composite restorations: a 10-year report. J Oral Rehabil 2004; 31:991–1000
3. Opdam N, Loomans B, Roeters F, Bronkhorst E. Five-year clinical performance of posterior resin composite restorations placed by dental students. J Dent 2004; 32:379–383
4. Van Meerbeek B, Vargas M, Inoue S, Yoshida Y, Peumans M, Lambrechts P et al. Adhesives and cements to promote preservation dentistry. Oper Dent 2001; 6:119–144
5. Yoshida Y, Nagakane K, Fukuda R, Nakayama Y, Okazaki M, Shintani H et al. Comparative study on adhesive performance of functional monomers. J Dent Res 2004; 83:454–458
6. Hobson R, McCabe J, Hogg S. Bond strength to surface enamel for different tooth types. Dent Mater 2001; 17:184–189
7. Yoshiyama M, Carvalho R, Sano H, Horner J, Brewer P, Pashley D. Interfacial morphology and strength of bonds made to superficial versus deep dentin. Am J Dent 1995; 8:297–302
8. Yoshiyama M, Carvalho R, Sano H, Horner J, Brewer P, Pashley D. Regional bond strengths of resins to human root dentine. J Dent 1996; 24:435–442
9. Yoshiyama M, Matsuo T, Ebisu S, Pashley D. Regional bond strengths of self-etching/self-priming adhesive systems. J Dent 1998; 26:609–616
10. Phrukkanon S, Burrow M, Tyas M. The effect of dentine location and tubule orientation on the bond strengths between resin and dentine. J Dent 1999; 27:265–274
11. Sattabanasuk V, Shimada Y, Tagami J. The bond of resin to different dentin surface characteristics. Oper Dent 2004; 29:333–341
12. Tay F, Pashley D. Resin bonding to cervical sclerotic dentin: a review. J Dent 2004; 32:173–196
13. Kusunoki M, Itoh K, Hisamitsu H, Wakumoto S. The efficacy of dentine adhesive to sclerotic dentine. J Dent 2002; 30:91–97
14. Kwong S, Cheung G, Kei L, Itthagarun A, Smales R, Tay F et al. Micro-tensile bond strengths to sclerotic dentin using a self-etching and a total-etching technique. Dent Mater 2002; 18:359–369
15. Kwong S, Tay F, Yip H, Kei L, Pashley D. An ultrastructural study of the application of dentine adhesives to acid-conditioned sclerotic dentine. J Dent 2000; 28:515–528
16. Van Meerbeek B, De Munck J, Mattar D, Van Landuyt K, Lambrechts P. Microtensile bond strengths of an etch&rinse and self-etch adhesive to enamel and dentin as a function of surface treatment. Oper Dent 2003; 28:647–660
17. Yazici A, Ozgunaltay G, Dayangac B. A scanning electron microscopic study of different caries removal techniques on human dentin. Oper Dent 2002; 27:360–366
18. Lussi A, Gygax M. Iatrogenic damage to adjacent teeth during classical approximal box preparation. J Dent 1998; 26:435–441
19. DeGrange M, Roulet F. Minimally invasive restorations with bonding. Quintessence, Chicago, 1997
20. Tyas M, Anusavice K, Frencken J, Mount G. Minimal intervention dentistry – a review. FDI Commission Project 1-97. Int Dent J 2000; 50:1–12
21. Murdoch-Kinch C, McLean M. Minimally invasive dentistry. J Am Dent Assoc 2003; 134:87–95
22. Burnett LJ, Conceicao E, Pelinos J, Eduardo C. Comparative study of influence on tensile bond strength of a composite to dentin using Er:YAG laser, air abrasion, or air turbine for preparation of cavities. J Clin Laser Med Surg 2001; 19:199–202
23. Gwinnett A. Smear layer: morphological considerations. Oper Dent Suppl 1984; 3:2–12
24. Blomlof J, Blomlof L, Lindskog S. Smear layer formed by different root planing modalities and its removal by an ethylenediaminetetraacetic acid gel preparation. Int J Periodon Restor Dent 1997; 17:242–249
25. Pashley D, Tao L, Boyd L, King G, Horner J. Scanning electron microscopy of the substructure of smear layers in human dentine. Arch Oral Biol 1988; 33:265–270

26. Prati C. Mechanisms of dentin bonding. Katholieke Universiteit, Leuven, Belgium, 1993, pp 171–191
27. Tani C, Finger W. Effect of smear layer thickness on bond strength mediated by three all-in-one self-etching priming adhesives. J Adhes Dent 2002; 4:283–289
28. Ruse N, Smith D. Adhesion to bovine dentin-surface characterization. J Dent Res 1991; 70:1002–1008
29. White G, Beech D, Tyas M. Dentin smear layer: an asset or a liability for bonding? Dent Mater 1989; 5:379–383
30. Clark-Holke D, Drake D, Walton R, Rivera E, Guthmiller J. Bacterial penetration through canals of endodontically treated teeth in the presence or absence of the smear layer. J Dent 2003; 31:275–281
31. Pashley D. Smear layer: physiological considerations. Oper Dent Suppl 1984; 3:13–29
32. Pashley D. Smear layer: overview of structure and function. Proc Finn Dent Soc Suppl 1992; 88:215–224
33. Pashley D. Clinical correlations of dentin structure and function. J Prosthet Dent 1991; 66:777–781
34. Tao L, Pashley D. Shear bond strengths to dentin: effects of surface treatments, depth and position. Dent Mater 1988; 4:371–378
35. Pashley D, Carvalho R. Dentine permeability and dentine adhesion. J Dent 1997; 25:355–372
36. Van Meerbeek B, De Munck J, Yoshida Y, Inoue S, Vargas M, Vijay P et al. Buonocore memorial lecture. Adhesion to enamel and dentin: current status and future challenges. Oper Dent 2003; 28:215–235
37. Pashley D. Dentin bonding: overview of the substrate with respect to adhesive material. J Esthet Dent 1991; 3:46–50
38. Pashley D, Michelich V, Kehl T. Dentin permeability: effects of smear layer removal. J Prosthet Dent 1981; 46:531–537
39. Pashley D. Dentin: a dynamic substrate – a review. Scanning Microsc 1989; 3:161–174
40. Tagami J, Tao L, Pashley D, Hosoda H, Sano H. Effects of high-speed cutting on dentin permeability and bonding. Dent Mater 1991; 7:234–239
41. Prati C, Pashley D, Montanari G. Hydrostatic intrapulpal pressure and bond strength of bonding systems. Dent Mater 1991; 7:54–58
42. Jacobsen T, Soderholm K. Some effects of water on dentin bonding. Dent Mater 1995; 11: 132–136
43. Shirai K, De Munck J, Yoshida Y et al. Effect of Cavity Configuration and aging on the bonding effectiveness of six adhesives to dentin. Dent Mater 2004; 21:110–124
44. Hirata K, Nakashima M, Sekine I, Mukouyama Y, Kimura K. Dentinal fluid movement associated with loading of restorations. J Dent Res 1991; 70:975–978
45. Tay F, Pashley D. Aggressiveness of contemporary self-etching systems. I: Depth of penetration beyond dentin smear layers. Dent Mater 2001; 17:296–308
46. Unemori M, Matsuya Y, Akashi A, Goto Y, Akamine A. Composite resin restoration and postoperative sensitivity: clinical follow-up in an undergraduate program. J Dent 2001; 29:7–13
47. Camps J, Dejou J, Remusat M, About I. Factors influencing pulpal response to cavity restorations. Dent Mater 2000; 16:432–440
48. Calt S, Serper A. Time-dependent effects of EDTA on dentin structures. J Endod 2002; 28:17–19
49. White G, Beech D, Tyas M. Dentin smear layer: an asset or a liability for bonding? Dent Mater 1989; 5:379–383
50. Inoue S, Van Meerbeek B, Abe Y, Yoshida Y, Lambrechts P, Vanherle G et al. Effect of remaining dentin thickness and the use of conditioner on micro-tensile bond strength of a glass-ionomer adhesive. Dent Mater 2001; 17:445–455
51. Bogra P, Kaswan S. Etching with EDTA an in vitro study. J Indian Soc Pedod Prev Dent 2003; 21:79–83
52. Viswanath D, Hegde A, Munshi A. The removal of the smear layer using EGTA: a scanning electron microscopic study. J Clin Pediatr Dent 2003; 28:69–74

53. Koibuchi H, Yasuda N, Nakabayashi N. Bonding to dentin with a self-etching primer: the effect of smear layers. Dent Mater 2001; 17:122–126
54. Opdam N, Roeters J, van Berghem E, Eijsvogels E, Bronkhorst E. Microleakage and damage to adjacent teeth when finishing class II adhesive preparations using either a sonic device or bur. Am J Dent 2002; 15:317–320
55. Wicht M, Haak R, Fritz U, Noack M. Primary preparation of class II cavities with oscillating systems. Am J Dent 2002; 15:21–25
56. Pioch T, Garcia-Godoy F, Duschner H, Koch M, Staehle H, Dorfer C. Effect of cavity preparation instruments (oscillating or rotating) on the composite–dentin interface in primary teeth. Dent Mater 2003; 19:259–263
57. Setien V, Cobb D, Denehy G, Vargas M. Cavity preparation devices: effect on microleakage of class V resin-based composite restorations. Am J Dent 2001; 14:157–162
58. Malmstrom H, Chaves Y, Moss M. Patient preference: conventional rotary handpieces or air abrasion for cavity preparation. Oper Dent 2003; 28:667–671
59. Mattar Lima D. Air abrasion: exploring its potential. Katholieke Universiteit, Leuven, Belgium, 2002
60. Geitel B, Kostka E, Wischnewski R, Roulet J. Tensile bond strength of composite to air-abraded enamel. J Adhes Dent 1999; 1:25–30
61. Borsatto M, Catirse A, Palma Dibb R, Nascimento T, Rocha R, Corona S. Shear bond strength of enamel surface treated with air-abrasive system. Braz Dent J 2002; 13:175–178
62. Mehl A, Kremers L, Salzmann K, Hickel R. 3D volume-ablation rate and thermal side effects with the Er:YAG and Nd:YAG laser. Dent Mater 1997; 13:246–251
63. Kawaguchi F, Eduardo C, Matos A. Nd:YAG laser influence on microleakage of class V composite restoration. J Clin Laser Med Surg 2003; 21:227–229
64. Attrill D, Davies R, King T, Dickinson M, Blinkhorn A. Thermal effects of the Er:YAG laser on a simulated dental pulp: a quantitative evaluation of the effects of a water spray. J Dent 2004; 32:35–40
65. Kataumi M, Nakajima M, Yamada T, Tagami J. Tensile bond strength and SEM evaluation of Er:YAG laser irradiated dentin using dentin adhesive. Dent Mater J 1998; 17:125–138
66. Ceballos L, Osorio R, Toledano M, Marshall G. Microleakage of composite restorations after acid or Er-YAG laser cavity treatments. Dent Mater 2001; 17:340–346
67. Ceballos L, Toledano M, Osorio R, Tay F, Marshall G. Bonding to Er-YAG-laser-treated dentin. J Dent Res 2002; 81:119–122
68. Ceballos L, Camejo D, Victoria F, Osorio R, Toledano M, Carvalho R et al. Microtensile bond strength of total-etch and self-etching adhesives to caries-affected dentine. J Dent 2003; 31:469–477
69. Armengol V, Laboux O, Weiss P, Jean A, Hamel H. Effects of Er:YAG and Nd:YAP laser irradiation on the surface roughness and free surface energy of enamel and dentin: an in vitro study. Oper Dent 2003; 28:67–74
70. Neev J, Stabholtz A, Liaw L, Torabinejad M, Fujishige J, Ho P et al. Scanning electron microscopy and thermal characteristics of dentin ablated by a short-pulse XeCl excimer laser. Lasers Surg Med 1993; 13:353–362
71. Visuri S, Gilbert J, Wright D, Wigdor H, Walsh JJ. Shear strength of composite bonded to Er:YAG laser-prepared dentin. J Dent Res 1996; 75:599–605
72. Kohara E, Hossain M, Kimura Y, Matsumoto K, Inoue M, Sasa R. Morphological and microleakage studies of the cavities prepared by Er:YAG laser irradiation in primary teeth. J Clin Laser Med Surg 2002; 20:141–147
73. Hossain M, Yamada Y, Nakamura Y, Murakami Y, Tamaki Y, Matsumoto K. A study on surface roughness and microleakage test in cavities prepared by Er:YAG laser irradiation and etched bur cavities. Lasers Med Sci 2003; 18:25–31
74. Martinez-Insua A, Da Silva D, Rivera F, Santana-Penin U. Differences in bonding to acid-etched or Er:YAG-laser-treated enamel and dentin surface. J Prosthet Dent 2000; 84:280–288
75. De Munck J, Van Meerbeek B, Yudhira R, Lambrechts P, Vanherle G. Micro-tensile bond strength of two adhesives to Erbium:YAG-lased vs bur-cut enamel and dentin. Eur J Oral Sci 2002; 110:322–329

76. Giachetti L, Russo D, Scarpelli F, Vitale M. SEM analysis of dentin treated with the Er:YAG laser: a pilot study of the consequences resulting from laser use on adhesion mechanisms. J Clin Laser Med Surg 2004; 22:35–41
77. Kameyama A, Kawada E, Amagai T, Takizawa M, Oda Y, Hirai Y. Effect of HEMA on bonding of Er:YAG laser-irradiated bovine dentine and 4-META/MMA-TBB resin. J Oral Rehabil 2002; 29:749–755
78. Gonzalez B, Ruiz P, Rodriguez N, Martin B, Varela P, Magan M et al. A comparative study of microleakage through enamel and cementum after laser Er:YAG instrumentation in class V cavity obturations, using scanning electron microscopy. J Clin Laser Med Surg 2002; 20: 197–201
79. Souza A de, Corona S, Palma Dibb R, Borsatto M, Pecora J. Influence of Er:YAG laser on tensile bond strength of a self-etching system and a flowable resin in different dentin depths. J Dent 2004; 32:269–275
80. Van Meerbeek B, Perdigão J, Lambrechts P, Vanherle G. The clinical performance of adhesives. J Dent 1998; 26:1–20
81. Nakabayashi N, Kojima K, Masuhara E. The promotion of adhesion by the infiltration of monomers into tooth substrates. J Biomed Mater Res 1982; 16:265–273
82. Tay F, Pashley D. Have dentin adhesives become too hydrophilic? J Can Dent Assoc 2003; 69:726–731
83. Van Meerbeek B, Inokoshi S, Braem M, Lambrechts P, Vanherle G. Morphological aspects of the resin-dentin interdiffusion zone with different dentin adhesive systems. J Dent Res 1992; 71:1530–1540
84. Van Meerbeek B, Conn L Jr, Duke E, Eick J, Robinson S, Guerrero D. Correlative transmission electron microscopy examination of nondemineralized and demineralized resin–dentin interfaces formed by two dentin adhesive systems. J Dent Res 1996; 75:879–888
85. Perdigão J, Lambrechts P, Van Meerbeek B, Braem M, Yildiz E, Yucel T et al. The interaction of adhesive systems with human dentin. Am J Dent 1996; 9:167–173
86. Ferrari M, Goracci G, Garcia-Godoy F. Bonding mechanism of three "one-bottle" systems to conditioned and unconditioned enamel and dentin. Am J Dent 1997; 10:224–230
87. Maciel K, Carvalho R, Ringle R, Preston C, Russell C, Pashley D. The effects of acetone, ethanol, HEMA, and air on the stiffness of human decalcified dentin matrix. J Dent Res 1996; 75:1851–1888
88. El Feninat F, Ellis T, Sacher E, Stangel I. A tapping mode AFM study of collapse and denaturation in dentinal collagen. Dent Mater 2001; 17:284–288
89. Nakabayashi N, Takarada K. Effect of HEMA on bonding to dentin. Dent Mater 1992; 8:125–130
90. Carvalho R, Mendonca J, Santiago S, Silveira R, Garcia F, Tay F et al. Effects of HEMA/solvent combinations on bond strength to dentin. J Dent Res 2003; 82:597–601
91. Van Meerbeek B, Dhem A, Goret-Nicaise M, Braem M, Lambrechts P, Vanherle G. Comparative SEM and TEM examination of the ultrastructure of the resin–dentin interdiffusion zone. J Dent Res 1993; 72:495–501
92. Inoue S, Vargas M, Abe Y, Yoshida Y, Lambrechts P, Vanherle G et al. Microtensile bond strength of eleven contemporary adhesives to dentin. J Adhes Dent 2001; 3:237–245
93. Van Meerbeek B, Kanumilli P, De Munck J, Van Landuyt K, Lambrechts P, Peumans M. A randomized, controlled trial evaluating the three-year clinical effectiveness of two etch & rinse adhesives in cervical lesions. Oper Dent 2004; 29:376–385
94. van Dijken J. Clinical evaluation of three adhesive systems in class V non-carious lesions. Dent Mater 2000; 16:285–291
95. Inoue S, Vargas M, Abe Y, Yoshida Y, Lambrechts P, Vanherle G et al. Microtensile bond strength of eleven contemporary adhesives to enamel. Am J Dent 2003; 16:329–334
96. Finger W, Balkenhol M. Practitioner variability effects on dentin bonding with an acetone-based one-bottle adhesive. J Adhes Dent 1999; 1:311–314
97. Gwinnett A. Chemically conditioned dentin: a comparison of conventional and environmental scanning electron microscopy findings. Dent Mater 1994; 10:150–155

98. Sano H, Shono T, Takatsu T, Hosoda H. Microporous dentin zone beneath resin-impregnated layer. Oper Dent 1994; 19:59–64
99. Jacobsen T, Soderholm K, Garcea I, Mondragon E. Calcium leaching from dentin and shear bond strength after etching with phosphoric acid of different concentrations. Eur J Oral Sci 2000; 108:247–254
100. Finger W, Balkenhol M. Rewetting strategies for bonding to dry dentin with an acetone-based adhesive. J Adhes Dent 2000; 2:51–56
101. Frankenberger R, Kramer N, Petschelt A. Technique sensitivity of dentin bonding: effect of application mistakes on bond strength and marginal adaptation. Oper Dent 2000; 25: 324–330
102. Gwinnett A. Moist versus dry dentin: its effect on shear bond strength. Am J Dent 1992; 5:127–129
103. Kanca J III. Effect of resin primer solvents and surface wetness on resin composite bond strength to dentin. Am J Dent 1992; 5:213–215
104. Tay F, Gwinnett A, Pang K, Wei S. Resin permeation into acid-conditioned, moist, and dry dentin: a paradigm using water-free adhesive primers. J Dent Res 1996; 75:1034–1044
105. Tay F, Gwinnett J, Wei S. Micromorphological spectrum from overdrying to overwetting acid-conditioned dentin in water-free acetone-based, single-bottle primer/adhesives. Dent Mater 1996; 12:236–244
106. Tay F, Gwinnett J, Wei S. The overwet phenomenon in two-component acetone-based primers containing aryl amine and carboxylic acid monomers. Dent Mater 1997; 13:118–127
107. Tay F, Gwinnett A, Wei S. The overwet phenomenon: an optical, micromorphological study of surface moisture in the acid-conditioned, resin-dentin interface. Am J Dent 1996; 9:43–48
108. Toledano M, Osorio R, Leonardi G de , Rosales-Leal J, Ceballos L, Cabrerizo-Vilchez M. Influence of self-etching primer on the resin adhesion to enamel and dentin. Am J Dent 2001; 14:205–210
109. Hashimoto M, Ohno H, Endo K, Kaga M, Sano H, Oguchi H. The effect of hybrid layer thickness on bond strength: demineralized dentin zone of the hybrid layer. Dent Mater 2000; 16:406–411
110. Hashimoto M, Ohno H, Kaga M, Endo K, Sano H, Oguchi H. In vivo degradation of resin-dentin bonds in humans over 1 to 3 years. J Dent Res 2000; 79:1385–1391
111. Pioch T, Staehle H, Duschner H, Garcia-Godoy F. Nanoleakage at the composite–dentin interface: a review. Am J Dent 2001; 14:252–258
112. Nystrom G, Holtan J, Phelps R, Becker W, Anderson T. Temperature and humidity effects on bond strength of a dentinal adhesive. Oper Dent 1998; 23:138–143
113. Tay F, Carvalho R, Sano H, Pashley D. Effect of smear layers on the bonding of a self-etching primer to dentin. J Adhes Dent 2000; 2:99–116
114. Tay F, Sano H, Carvalho R, Pashley E, Pashley D. An ultrastructural study of the influence of acidity of self-etching primers and smear layer thickness on bonding to intact dentin. J Adhes Dent 2000b; 2:83–98
115. Inoue S, Van Meerbeek B, Vargas M, Yoshida Y, Lambrechts P, Vanherle G. Adhesion mechanisms of self-etching adhesives. Am J Dent 1999; 10:131–175
116. Frankenberger R, Perdigão J, Rosa B, Lopes M. "No-bottle" vs "multi-bottle" dentin adhesives: a microtensile bond strength and morphological study. Dent Mater 2001; 17:373–380
117. Chan K, Tay F, King N, Imazato S, Pashley D. Bonding of mild self-etching primers/adhesives to dentin with thick smear layers. Am J Dent 2003; 16:340–346
118. Watanabe I, Nakabayashi N, Pashley D. Bonding to ground dentin by a phenyl-P self-etching primer. J Dent Res 1994; 73:1212–1220
119. De Munck J, Van Meerbeek B, Vargas M et al. One day bonding effectiveness of new self-etch adhesives to bur-cut enamel and dentin. Oper Dent (in press)
120. De Munck J. An in vitro and in vivo study on the durability of biomaterial-tooth bonds: Katholieke Universiteit, Leuven, Belgium, 2004
121. Oliveira S, Marshall S, Hilton J, Marshall G. Etching kinetics of a self-etching primer. Biomaterials 2002; 23:4105–4112

122. Yoshida Y, Van Meerbeek B, Nakayama Y, Snauwaert J, Hellemans L, Lambrechts P et al. Evidence of chemical bonding at biomaterial-hard tissue interfaces. J Dent Res 2000; 79: 709–714
123. Tay F, King N, Chan K, Pashley D. How can nanoleakage occur in self-etching adhesive systems that demineralize and infiltrate simultaneously? J Adhes Dent 2002; 4:255–269
124. Turkun S. Clinical evaluation of a self-etching and a one-bottle adhesive system at two years. J Dent 2003; 31:527–534
125. Peumans M, Van Meerbeek B, De Munck J, Lambrechts P. Two-year clinical effectiveness of a self-etch adhesive in cervical lesions. Oper Dent (in press)
126. Peumans M, Kanumilli P, De Munck J, Van Landuyt K, Lambrechts P, Van Meerbeek B. Clinical effectiveness of contemporary adhesives: a review of current clinical trials. Dent Mater 2005
127. Cho B, Dickens S. Effects of the acetone content of single solution dentin bonding agents on the adhesive layer thickness and the microtensile bond strength. Dent Mater 2004; 20: 107–115
128. Haller B. Recent developments in dentin bonding. Am J Dent 2000; 13:44–50
129. Walker M, Wang Y, Swafford J, Evans A, Spencer P. Influence of additional acid etch treatment on resin cement dentin infiltration. J Prosthodont 2000; 9:77–81
130. Agee K, Pashley E, Itthagarun A, Sano H, Tay F, Pashley D. Submicron hiati in acid-etched dentin are artifacts of desiccation. Dent Mater 2003; 19:60–68
131. Carvalho R, Chersoni S, Frankenberger R, Pashley D, Prati C, Tay F. A challenge to the conventional wisdom that simultaneous etching and resin infiltration always occurs in self-etch adhesives. Biomaterials 2005; 26:1035–1042
132. Itthagarun A, Tay F. Self-contamination of deep dentin by dentin fluid. Am J Dent 2000; 13:195–200
133. Perdigão J, Geraldeli S, Hodges J. Total-etch versus self-etch adhesive: effect on postoperative sensitivity. J Am Dent Assoc 2003; 132:1621–1629
134. Fritz U, Finger W. Bonding efficiency of single-bottle enamel/dentin adhesives. Am J Dent 1999; 12:277–282
135. Bouillaguet S, Gysi P, Wataha J, Ciucchi B, Cattani M, Godin C et al. Bond strength of composite to dentin using conventional, one-step, and self-etching adhesive systems. J Dent 2001; 29:55–61
136. Tay F, Pashley D. Permeability of single-step, self-etch adhesives: the cost of saving time. Tokyo, 2001, pp 23–39
137. Tay F, Pashley D, Suh B, Carvalho R, Itthagarun A. Single-step adhesives are permeable membranes. J Dent 2002; 30:371–82
138. Tay F, Pashley D, Yoshiyama M. Two modes of nanoleakage expression in single-step adhesives. J Dent Res 2002; 81:472–476
139. De Munck J, Van Meerbeek B, Yoshida Y, Inoue S, Vargas M, Suzuki K et al. Four-year water degradation of total-etch adhesives bonded to dentin. J Dent Res 2003; 82:136–140
140. Hashimoto M, Tay F, Ohno H, Sano H, Kaga M, Yiu C et al. SEM and TEM analysis of water degradation of human dentinal collagen. J Biomed Mater Res 2003; 66B:287–298
141. Tay F, Pashley D. Water treeing: a potential mechanism for degradation of dentin adhesives. Am J Dent 2003; 16:6–12
142. Van Landuyt K, De Munck J, Snauwaert J et al. Phase-separation in contemporary one-step self-etch adhesives. J Dent Res 2005; 84:183–188
143. Yoshida Y, Van Meerbeek B, Nakayama Y, Yoshioka M, Snauwaert J, Abe Y et al. Adhesion to and decalcification of hydroxyapatite by carboxylic acids. J Dent Res 2001; 80:1565–1569
144. Yoshioka M, Yoshida Y, Inoue S, Lambrechts P, Vanherle G, Nomura Y et al. Adhesion/decalcification mechanisms of acid interactions with human hard tissues. J Biomed Mater Res 2002; 59:56–62
145. Van Meerbeek B, Yoshida Y, Inoue S et al. Interfacial characteristics of resin-modified glass-ionomers bonded to dentin. J Dent Res 2001; 80

146. Folwaczny M, Mehl A, Kunzelmann K, Hickel R. Clinical performance of a resin-modified glass-ionomer and a compomer in restoring non-carious cervical lesions: 5-year results. Am J Dent 2001; 14:153–156
147. Tyas M, Burrow M. Clinical evaluation of a resin-modified glass ionomer adhesive system: results at five years. Oper Dent 2002; 27:438–441
148. Kanumilli P. Clinical and laboratory effectiveness of contemporary adhesives. Katholieke Universiteit, Leuven, Belgium, 2004

In Situ Photo-Polymerisation and Polymerisation-Shrinkage Phenomena 6

D. Watts, N. Silikas

Introduction

Photo-polymerisation is now a widely accepted initiation mode for the clinical hardening processes required with a wide range of biomaterials including dental adhesives and restoratives. As we discuss in detail, there is a strong relationship between the progressive phenomenon of photo-polymerisation, with attendant network formation, and shrinkage stresses and strains set up in the material and its host environment. Molecular densification during the polymerisation process of dental restoratives, and the macroscopic effects of shrinkage strain and/or shrinkage stress, continue to attract widespread international research interest [1–13]. This is pursued at several levels. There is the need to characterise these properties of both candidate monomer molecules, synthesised with the aim of attaining reduced shrinkage materials [14], and also resin-composite materials – either commercially available or formulated experimentally [10]. In addition, different light-curing units and modes of operation require investigation with representative materials in the context of shrinkage phenomena [3, 15, 16]. These properties are strongly coupled and are controlled especially by the *degree of conversion* (*DC*) of the network [3]; thus, there are numerous variables associated with the photo-polymerisation process, and an understanding of these is important for the dentist and the dental scientist.

Potential Clinical Consequences of Shrinkage Phenomena

Several clinical factors are often discussed in relation to polymerisation shrinkage phenomena. These factors are often arranged in a causal sequence, with shrinkage being seen as the underlying root cause; however, this is evidently an oversimplified model, since multiple causes can contribute to problems such as micro-leakage, debonding and especially post-operative pain. Nevertheless, shrinkage is one crucial factor in relation to several clinical outcomes.

The objective of this chapter is not to exhaustively review the clinical evidence but to discuss the underlying science of shrinkage behaviour, in its dependence upon photo-polymerisation.

Marginal Staining

Marginal staining is often the first indicator that the clinician sees some possible breakdown or aesthetic deficiency of a restoration. This is not necessarily a sign of any serious problem meriting replacement of the restoration for any functional or biological reason; however, such staining does show that at least superficial deterioration has occurred at the margin. Stresses caused by shrinkage effects are a probable cause.

Fractures

When restorations in a host cavity develop internal stresses, this is a pre-disposing factor in material fracture, especially in the restorative material itself; however, the shrinkage stresses most probably operate in concert with stresses due to occlusion and even due to intra-oral thermal changes.

Debonding

It is well documented that teeth deform under the cinfluence of externally applied loads [17]. Similarly, cuspal deflection due to internal shrinkage stresses has been reported. Various techniques indicated cuspal deflections of up to 50 µm. Deformation of the tooth depends on the distribution of the residual stresses; hence, tooth deformations may take a range of values. Deformation patterns have been studied using numerical techniques, such as finite element analysis [2, 18, 19].

Microleakage

If debonding has occurred and if a gap also results, this may lead to leakage at the gaps, including ingress of bacteria.

Secondary Caries

Although secondary caries is a major factor in restoration failure, it should be remembered that this is a feature of many kinds of restorative techniques other than those that undergo polymerisation; hence, polymerisation shrinkage is unlikely to be the sole cause of secondary caries with resin-composite restorations.

Postoperative Pain

Several myths are often repeated about resin composites "shrinking towards the light" and hence pulling away from the floor of a cavity. That composite materials exhibit gaps at the pulpal floor, and that shrinkage may have a contributory role, may nevertheless be probable. This void eventually fills with fluid and can cause hydrostatic pressure in the dentinal tubules, which leads to sensitivity to pressure on the filling. This is the most common reason for pain when biting on a new composite filling. The only solution for this problem is to redo the filling [20, 21]; however, an inevitable causal link between shrinkage and post-operative pain should be doubted.

Clinical Management of Shrinkage Phenomena

Shrinkage stresses are very dependent upon the cavity geometry as well as the underlying chemistry. This is often helpfully discussed in terms of C-factor, the ratio of bonded to unbonded surface area of the restoration. There may be opportunities in cavity design to adjust the shape so as to suitably modify the C-factor and the resultant stress.

It is clinically possible to reduce composite curing rate by lowering the light irradiance used for photo-activation. In one model for reaction kinetics, conversion rate is proportional to the square root of the irradiance (in mW/cm^2); however, to be effective, these new "soft-start" curing methods should be able to reduce shrinkage stress, or at least the shrinkage-stress rate, and improve marginal integrity significantly, without compromising the *DC* or composite mechanical properties.

Light Sources for Photo-Polymerisation of Dental Biomaterials

Understanding photo-polymerisation begins with an understanding of light itself. Since the time of Isaac Newton, the wave and particle models of light were in competition until the Quantum revolution of the early twentieth century, when these models were combined in the quantum synthesis. In our discussion related to photochemistry, it is helpful to highlight the particle, or photon, model.

Photons, the particles of light, have several characteristics:

1. Energy (frequency, wavelength) and its distribution. The energy of a photon of frequency ν is given by $E=h\nu$, where h is Planck's constant. Because the energy of photons is directly proportional to their frequency, low-energy photons have low frequencies, while high-energy photons have high frequencies. Low-energy photons are called radiowaves or microwaves, medium-energy photons are called light (or light waves, or visible light), high-energy photons are called X-rays, and those having even higher energy are called gamma rays.
2. Momentum. The momentum of a photon is given by dividing the energy by the speed of light.
3. Number/area/second (expressed equivalently as irradiance).
4. Spin (polarisation). In quantum mechanics, spin is an intrinsic angular momentum associated with particles. Photons should be observed in three spin projections (−1, 0 and 1); however, the zero projection would require a frame where the photon is at rest, but, since photons travel at the speed of light, such a frame does not exist according to the theory of relativity, and so photons only have two spin projections.

5. Entanglement. Photon entanglement is a quantum phenomenon that occurs when two or more photons share unique properties but remain physically separated.

Photons may be produced by several different types of light source. These sources include: quartz–tungsten–halogen (QTH); plasma arc; laser; and light-emitting diode (LED).

Quartz–Tungsten–Halogen Sources

A quartz–tungsten–halogen light source consists of a halogen bulb with a filament. As a current passes through the filament, the wire heats up, and as a result, electromagnetic radiation is emitted from the filament [22]. The traditional standard irradiance of the QTH sources has been approximately 500 mW/cm^2, which can adequately cure most dental composites to a depth of 2 mm in approximately 40 s. The spectrum of QTH radiation is continuous over the visible range, with radiation intensity increasing considerably towards the red end of the spectrum. Most of this radiation does not contribute to polymerisation and must be filtered [23]. The QTH sources require filters to select blue-light wavelengths between approximately 400 and 500 nm.

Plasma Arc Curing Sources

Plasma arc curing (PAC) sources contain xenon plasma lamps. The light is emitted from glowing plasma, which is composed of a gaseous mixture of ionised molecules and electrons. The lamp filled with high-pressure xenon gas emits high-intensity light by an electric discharge. They are characterised by a very high output in a narrow range of wavelengths around 470 nm [24]. Their claim is that the higher the light intensity, the higher penetration depth is achieved in a short time by these systems; however, this raises the question of whether the high irradiance delivered in short time would lead to an adequate polymerisation. Another issue of concern is the rate of polymerisation. Curing by PAC sources occurs very fast and there is the risk of high polymerisation shrinkage.

Laser Sources

Laser sources emit light at a few distinct frequencies within the desired region, thus completely eliminating the need for filtering undesired wavelengths. AccuCure-3000 is a commercially developed Laser-LCU whose output spectrum falls entirely within the absorption spectrum of CQ. A study by Blankenau has shown that the AccuCure-3000 produced post cure physical characteristics that are much improved over those attained by an Argon-Ion laser and QTH light sources [25].

Light-Emitting-Diode Sources

Light-emitting-diode sources are semi-conductor devices of an n–p type, constructed from two layers of semi-conducting materials, one doped with electrons (n-doped), the other doped with "holes" (p-type). The ends of the crystals are cleaved and polished to give a laser resonant cavity (the ends rarely necessitate reflective coatings). When a small voltage is applied to the terminals, electrons are injected from the n-region into the p-region (and the holes from p- to n-region). The holes and electrons rejoin emitting photons of identical wavelengths. This recombinant radiation forms the basis for the LED and explains the narrow bandwidth of the light emitted [26]. The wavelength of the emitted light is not only dependent on the crystal structure – in the case of the blue diode it is gallium-nitride (GaN) – but also on the length and refractive index of the semi-conductor crystal [27]. GaN LEDs were first proposed for activation of dental light-cured composites by Mills [28] in a letter to the editor of the "British Dental Journal". Individual LEDs have a relatively low light irradiance output compared with a QTH bulb; therefore, multiple diodes are often arranged into an array, the combined output of which, when appropriately channelled through a light guide, can approach that of QTH values [29]. Spectral output of one QTH source (Optilux 501) and two LED sources (Freelight-1 and Ultralume-2) are shown in Fig. 6.1.

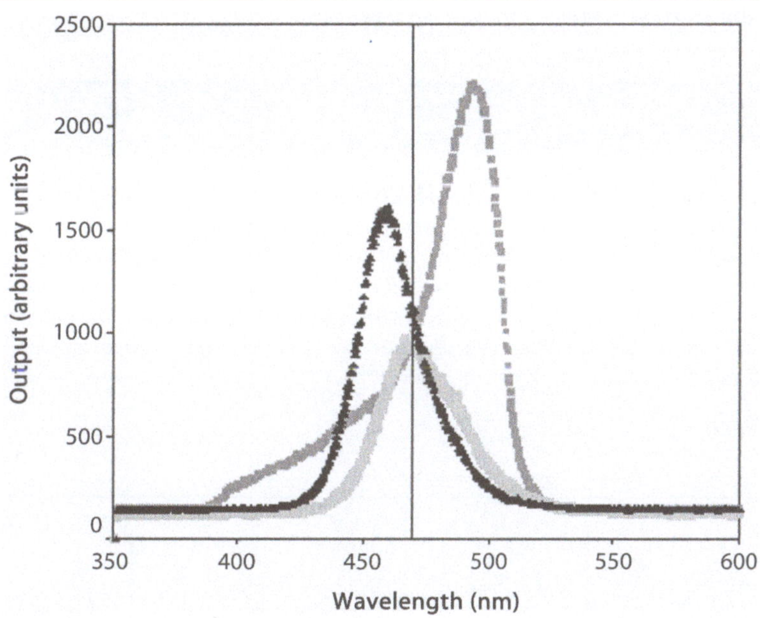

Fig. 6.1. Spectral output of one quartz–tungsten–halogen source (Optilux 501) and two light-emitting diode sources (Freelight-1 and Ultralume-2)

Further Variables with Light Sources

Alternative curing routines using stepped, pulsed or ramped energy delivery have been developed with the intent of improving restoration interfacial integrity by reducing composite curing rate, thereby increasing its flow capacity. A slow polymerisation of a resin composite may give rise to reduced polymerisation shrinkage in restorations because of stress relief. This may be achieved by applying short pulses of light energy (pulsed delay), pre-polymerisation at low light intensity followed by final exposure at high intensity (soft start), or a combination of both (ramp curing).

In pulse-delay cure the polymerisation is initiated by a short flash of light followed by a waiting time of several minutes before the final polymerisation is performed. It was shown that pulse activation and soft-start polymerisation regimens did not significantly reduce post-gel shrinkage [30], and that pulse-delay technique resulted in a polymer structure with lower crosslink density compared with slow-start polymerisation [31].

The soft start was found to reduce the speed of shrinkage while maintaining degree of cure [3, 32]. Other potential benefits of soft start include reduced polymerisation shrinkage and temperature rising [33], lower solubility and equivalent hardness values compared with a standard halogen source [34].

The ramped light intensity can slow the rate of cure and help to reduce the rate and maximum polymerisation stress without compromising the physical properties of the material [35].

Radiometry: Irradiance (Radiant Incidence and Radiant Exitance) and Total Energy Concept

Irradiance is a term that can legitimately be used for light output from a source and also for light input onto a defined surface area; thus, there are two possible conditions. The flux can be arriving at the surface (Fig. 6.2 a), in which case the radiant flux density – or optical power received per unit area on the surface – may also be referred to uniquely as radiant incidence. The flux can arrive from any direction above the surface, as indicated by the rays. Irradiance in this case is defined as:

$$M = d\Phi/dA$$

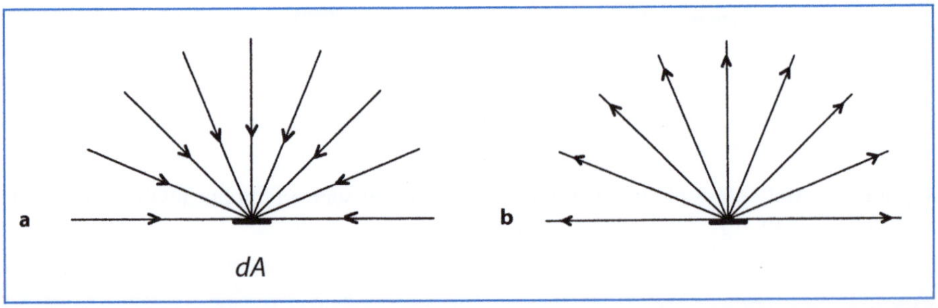

Fig. 6.2. **a** Radiant incidence; **b** radiant exitance

where Φ is the radiant flux arriving at the point and dA is the differential area surrounding the point.

The flux can also be leaving the surface due to emission and/or reflection (Fig. 6.2b). The radiant flux density is then referred to as radiant exitance. The flux can leave in any direction above the surface. Irradiance in this case is defined as:

$$E = d\Phi/dA$$

where Φ is the radiant flux leaving the point and dA is the differential area surrounding the point.

Since irradiance is equivalent to power (or energy/time) per unit area, then the integral of irradiance and time is equivalent to total energy per unit area. In cases where the irradiance is constant over a time interval, then the product of the irradiance and time gives the value of the total-energy integral. This parameter is often used when investigating the dependence of photo-polymerisation upon irradiation conditions.

Light Penetration into and Through Oral Biomaterials

Depth of Cure, and Top/Bottom Surface Hardness

A major characteristic of visible light-cured (VLC) composites is the variable depth of cure, which arises from attenuation of light transmission in these materials. The variation of cure with depth into composite filling materials has been studied by several techniques, including microhardness profiles [36, 37] and *DC* [38]. Several techniques have been compared [39–41].

Several parameters may be derived to characterise the depth of cure; these include the depth at which hardness falls to 80% of its peak value [37] and the depth at which the hardness falls to the lowest measurable value [42]. A resin which is not fully polymerised will show reduced mechanical properties, poorer colour stability and greater susceptibility to stain.

With the development of light sources of improved irradiance, at least a 2- to 3-mm depth of material can be polymerised in 20–30 s irradiation. Irradiance falls within the body of the material because of absorption and scattering by the resin and filler particles, and by tooth substance.

Surface Reflection, Absorption and Scattering Processes in Composites

Aesthetic restorative materials should match the optical properties of hard dental tissues, especially in colour and translucency. The colour of the composites reflects the reflectance spectrum (i.e. light reflection) of the composites, which are considerably affected by the background colour and the thickness of the composites [43].

According to Fresnel's relationship, for light incident to a normal plane boundary between media of refractive index n_1 and n_2, the reflectance [r] is:

$$r = \frac{(n_1 - n_2)^2}{(n_1 + n_2)^2}$$

Hence, a composite is only translucent when there is matching of refractive indices between resin matrix and filler [44]. For methacrylate resins, the n is ~1.5. Adjustments in refractive index over a small range can be made by change in the ratio of primary and diluent monomers, such as Bis-GMA/TEGDMA. Of the glass fillers, n=1.552 at the peak wavelength, ca. 470 nm, for a widely used barium glass. Under the same conditions, n=1.506 for a strontium glass.

The theory of scattering is not well developed for particulate glass composite resins of the appropriate particle size ranges, volume fractions and refractive index increments (Δn). Rayleigh scattering describes the case where particles are small compared with wavelength, Rayleigh-Gans scattering applies to larger particles provided that Δn is small. The more general Mie theory is still not fully applicable and empirical relationships have been widely employed.

Kubelka and Munk (K-M) [45] mathematically expressed optical properties, such as light reflection and transmission of translucent light-scattering materials, in terms of simple hyperbolic functions of their thickness, dependent upon two optical constants such as absorption and scattering coefficients at each wavelength in the visible light spectrum. Because K-M's theory could successfully predict reflection spectra and colour of translucent light-scattering materials of differing thickness on various backgrounds, several dental materials scientists and clinicians have applied this theory to the evaluation of optical properties, especially light reflection, of set dental aesthetic restorative materials [43, 46–49]. There are, however, few studies of optical properties, especially light transmission, of uncured VL-cured composites by K-M's theory [48].

Composites may be provided in both opaque and translucent forms to match different areas of the dentition. Metallic pigments are added in small quantities to give different tints; these absorb rather than scatter light.

The optical properties of composites can change as a result of polymerisation. The extent of change is dependent upon the characteristics of the material and wavelength [50]. When VLC resins are cured, n_{resin} and hence Δn change slightly. This can produce a significant change in light transmission and appearance of the composite. The translucency can increase or decrease, depending upon whether $n_{resin} > n_{glass}$, or vice versa.

The camphoroquinone photo-sensitiser imparts a yellow tint to the monomers, which is lost as CQ is consumed. Residual amine-reducing agents may degrade in clinical service and cause discolouration of the composite.

Surface reflectivity and gloss depends strongly on the mean particle size. Polishable composites, which retain a gloss caused by specular reflection, are based on particle sizes ca. 0.5 µm. Colour matching of composites for use under artificial lighting, which may include UV components, is difficult.

Application of Beer-Lambert Law

Regarding the Beer-Lambert law, light is attenuated with increasing cross-sectional distance from the irradiated surface [51] as a result of light absorption and scattering caused by fillers and other additives [52], leading to limited depth of cure [37].

To express this mathematically, firstly, the relationships must be established between the light levels incident upon the surface and those available at depth within the specimen. This is given by the Lambert law:

$$I = I_0 e^{-\gamma d}$$

where I_o is the light intensity *entering* the specimen surface and I is the light intensity at depth d below the surface. γ is the Naperian absorption coefficient of the medium. Changing to a decadic exponent, the transmittance τ, which expresses the available light intensity within the medium at depth d, is defined as:

$$\tau = \frac{I}{I_0} = 10^{-\alpha} = 10^{-ad}$$

where α is the absorbance and γ=2.303x a. The (decadic) linear absorption coefficient [a] includes the effects of absorption by all components of the resin-composite system, as well as scattering effects. (If the camphorquinone concentration is unnecessarily high, this will lead to attenuation of radiation through the material.)

Secondly, the light intensity absorbed by the photo-sensitiser across a thickness element δd, at depth d in the medium, is then:

$$I_a = I.[1 - e^{-a_s \delta d}] \approx I.a_s \delta d$$

where a_s is the absorption coefficient of the photo-sensitiser. The value of $a_s \delta d$ is given by Beer's law:

$$a_s \delta d = \varepsilon_s \,.\, C_s$$

where ε_s is the molar absorptivity (extinction coefficient) of the photo-sensitiser [concentration C_S], at the particular frequency of radiation absorbed.

The overall expression for nonuniform monochromatic light absorption of the composite system, in terms of the number of quanta absorbed by the photo-sensitiser per unit volume at a distance d below the surface, may be given by:

$$I_a = \varepsilon_s C_s I_0 10^{-ad}$$

It may often suffice to assume that, at depth within the composite, the concentration C_S of the photo-sensitiser is constant, where this is present in excess of the photon intensity.

Photo-Initiators for Free-Radical and Cationic Polymerisation

Most VLC dental composites are supplied as single-component formulations. Resin composites formulated as dual-component types undergo either self-cure upon mixing, or dual cure upon mixing *and* application of visible light, i.e. dual-cure systems incorporate both self-cure and VLC activator/initiator chemicals. These are commonly, but improperly, denoted the "catalyst" system(s).

The organic monomer phase usually includes low concentrations of inhibitors and stabilisers together with the chemicals required for activation and initiation of monomer polymerisation or "cure". The initiation process has a significant effect on the kinetics of polymerisation and the polymer structure; thus, it can affect several properties, such as rheology and long-term performance, of the network. The structure of radicals and their effect on the rate of reaction is critical to the development of an understanding of polymerisation [53].

Camphorquinone

The VLC resin-composite materials usually employ photo-sensitised free-radical initiators, commonly, an α-1,2 diketone, such as benzyl or camphorquinone (CQ; Fig. 6.3), and an amine-reducing agent such as dimethylaminoethyl methacrylate (DMAEMA) or dimethyl p-toluidine (DMPTI) [54, 55].

The CQ/amine photo-initiator system for generating radicals is widely used for the polymerisation of dental restorative materials. Light is absorbed by CQ in the blue region and leads to the $n \rightarrow \pi^*$ transition of the dicarbonyl group [56]. The nonbonding electrons can be promoted to a π^* antibonding orbital. This excited state has a half-life of approximately 0.05 ms. The excited $n \rightarrow \pi^*$ transition interacts with an amine molecule and forms an exciplex, which is an excited short-lived state. Within this exciplex, CQ accepts an electron from amine and from the radical ion pair, and abstracts a hydrogen atom from the tertiary amine which results in the primary radical. This latter radical then attacks the carbon double bonds of the monomers. The former CQ radical may retard polymerisation through termination reactions [57].

The concentration of CQ photo-sensitiser is in the range 0.17–1.03 mass percent of the resin phase and that of DMAEMA reducing agent is 0.86–1.39 mass percent [55]. The combined photo-sensitiser/ reducing-agent complex has an extended absorption band within the VL spectrum.

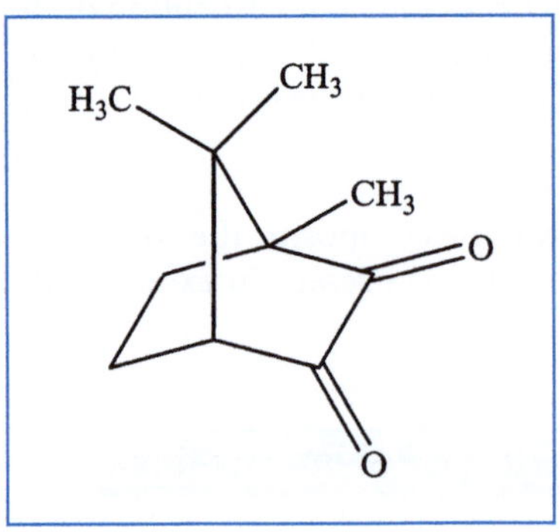

Fig. 6.3. Chemical structure of camphoroquinone (CQ)

1-Phenyl-1,2-propanedione

Camphorquinone is inherently yellow, which causes problems in colour matching. This, in turn, places practical limits on the concentration of CQ and, consequently, limits the degree of polymerisation and depth of cure that can be attained; therefore, alternative photo-sensitisers have been considered. Diacetyl (2,3-butanedione) and propanal have been studied by Peutzfeldt and Asmussen [58, 59]. A prominent initiator is 1-phenyl-1,2-propanedione (PPD) which has an aromatic group on one side of the dicarbonyl and a methyl group on the other (Fig. 6.4) and $\lambda_{max}\approx 410$ nm. Recent experiments showed that PPD would be an efficient visible light photo-sensitiser, comparable with camphorquinone, for the initiation of the dental resin polymerisation [60], and that resins initiated with PPD showed better mechanical properties than those initiated with CQ [61]. Furthermore, PPD can act synergistically with CQ to increase the monomer conversion to polymer and/or reduce the photo-sensitiser concentration (and, hence, colour). This blend of photo-sensitisers may produce a better balance between surface cure and bulk cure [62]. The combination will also contribute to a reduction in chroma (from deep yellow to a pale yellow) when the total photo-sensitiser (PPD+CQ) concentration is held constant since the PPD wavelength ($\lambda_{max}\approx 410$ nm) will shift the hue to a less yellow shade (shorter dominant wavelength). The absorption spectra of CQ+PPD is shown in Fig. 6.5.

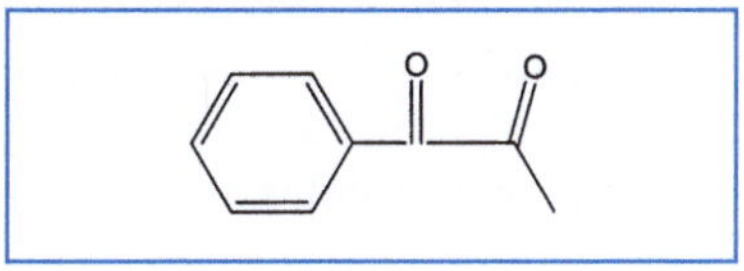

Fig. 6.4. Chemical structure of 1 phenyl 1,2 propanedione (PPD)

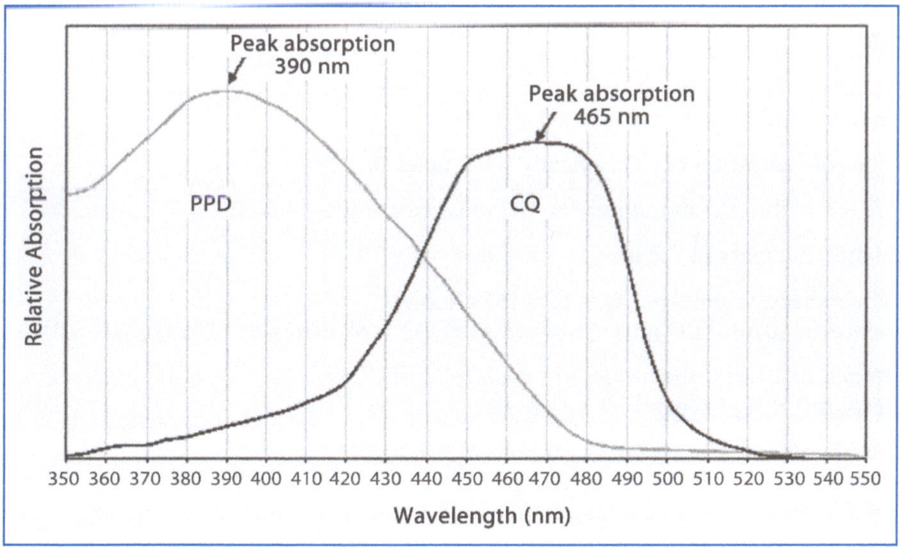

Fig. 6.5. Absorption spectra of CQ+PPD

Photon Numbers and Photo-Initiation

It is useful to calculate the typical numbers of photons produced by a light source per second and to compare this with the numbers of photoinitiator molecules commonly employed.

Regarding photons produced by a light source, the following terms and relationships are defined:

I = irradiance of light source (mW/cm^2), e.g. 500

λ = wavelength of light (nm), e.g. 470

υ = frequency of light (Hz)

c = velocity of light [3×10^8 m/s]

h = Planck's constant [6.626×10^{-34} J.s]

$E = h.\upsilon = h.c/\lambda$

E = energy of 1 photon of light = $4.226.10^{-1}$ J, for λ_{470}

N_{ph} = number of photons emitted per second and per square centimetre.

$N_{ph} = I/E = I$ [mW/cm^2 or $mJ/(s.cm^2)$/E [J]

Thus, for a typical blue light wavelength: λ_{470}

$N_{ph} = 1.185\times10^{18}.\ 1\times10^{18}$ photons/($s.cm^2$)

How many molecules of CQ are in a disk of monomer?

d = 5 mm
h = 2 mm
$A = \pi(2.5)^2 \approx 20\ mm^3$. $V = A.h = 40\ mm^3$.

If monomer density = 1.0 g/cm^3 = 0.001 g/mm^3,
then monomer mass = 0.001×40 = 0.04 g.

The concentration of CQ typically = 0.2 mass %.

Hence, within the monomer, the CQ mass fraction is $f = 0.002$.

Hence, the mass of CQ is $M_{CQ} = f \times 0.04 = 8 \times 10^{-5}$ g.

The molecular mass of CQ is **m** = 166 g/mole;
hence, in 40 mm^3 the number of moles of CQ = $M_{CQ}/\mathbf{m} = 8\times10^{-5}/166.\ 4.8\times10^{-7}$.

Hence, in 40 mm^3 the number of molecules of CQ =
($M_{CQ}/\mathbf{m}$) × N_A (Avogadro's number).

$= (4.8\times10^{-7}) \times (6.023\times10^{23}) = 0.289\times10^{18}\ 0.3\times10^{18}$

With a composite consisting of 30% monomer, the number of CQ molecules in a 40-mm^3 disc is calculated as follows:

$N_{CQ} = (0.3\times10^{18}) \times 0.3 = 0.09\times10^{18}\ 0.1\times10^{18}$

This is the CQ content, in a material thickness of 2 mm.
This can be compared with the number of photons supplies per second per 20 mm^2 disc area:

N_{ph} .0.2×10^{18} photons per second per 20 mm^2.

It is concluded that the number of photons arriving per second is comparable to the number of CQ molecules in the corresponding area or volume of the material.

Extent of Polymerisation

It is evident from many studies [63–66] that all of the dimethacrylate monomers exhibit considerable residual unsaturation in the final product. This ranges from 25 to 45 %, or *degree of conversion* (*DC*) ranging from 55 to 75 %. The nature of the unpolymerised resin is of considerable concern, especially in terms of deleterious effects on the mechanical properties and dimensional stability of the restoration, but less so in terms of biocompatibility [67]. The unconverted methacrylate groups must reside in the polymer network either as residual monomer or (a majority) as pendant side chains (PSC) which extend from the main chains by virtue of having reacted at only one end of the difunctional molecule. A further possibility is a cyclisation reaction. As residual monomer, these molecules function as plasticising agents which can reduce the properties of the polymer network. This occurs until such time as the monomers leach from the composite into the oral environment. Pendant side chains act as permanent plasticisers in the composite; hence, it is desirable to increase *DC* in order to produce stiffer and more durable resins, although, for a given composite, shrinkage increases with *DC*.

For a given VLC product the *DC* depends on the (a) light irradiance reaching the composite surface, (b) time of exposure and (c) thermal energy within the system.

The structure, composition and polarity of the diluent monomer molecules affects the *DC* and also shrinkage, water sorption and mechanical properties. The greater the proportion of BIS-GMA in the composite, the lower its *DC* [68–70].

Thermal and Spectroscopic Probes

Several techniques have been used to measure the extent of the reactions and to identify the formation of radicals.

Photo-DSC

Differential scanning calorimetry (DSC) can determine the rate of reaction and can be applied to the development of kinetic models. It has been used successfully to predict the incomplete polymerisation in commercial dental light-cured composites [71].

FTIR Spectroscopy

The unpolymerised carbon–carbon double bonds give rise to an infrared (IR) absorption at 1638 cm^{-1}, which enables determination of *DC* either by analysis of the filled composite, using multiple internal reflection IR, or by analysis of the unfilled resin films in transmission after extraction of the filler with a suitable organic solvent. The methods appear to provide comparable results for the same resin composites, although data suggest that *DC* is slightly reduced in composites containing large-volume fractions of quartz or barium glass [72].

Photo-polymerisation reactions occur very fast. Real-time FTIR is an experimental technique that offers the possibility to monitor these reactions in real time [73]. It offers adequate time resolution and analytic capabilities to study the kinetics of photo-polymerisation in situ [74].

NIR Spectroscopy

Near-infrared spectroscopy can measure Overton and combination bands of the C=C vibrations [75]. This has the capability of measuring relatively thick specimens.

FT-Raman

Raman spectroscopy offers an alternative to FTIR spectroscopy for evaluating the *DC* in dental resins and follows it at the early stages of polymerisation [76–78]. Raman spectroscopy can also be used to study the composition and structure of bonding of a sample [79, 80].

Solid-State NMR

Solid-state NMR has been used to measure the conversion of methacrylate resins [81, 82].

EPR Spectroscopy

During photo-polymerisation, radicals are generated from the CQ/amine exciplex and these in turn generate radicals on the growing polymer chains. The former radicals are unlikely to have an extended lifetime, but the polymer radicals may be expected to persist for some time after the apparent cessation of polymerisation following the vitrification of the resin-composite mass. The presence and lifetime of free radicals may be detected by electron paramagnetic resonance (EPR) spectroscopy [83]. In other cases, radicals have been detected with much longer lifetimes. The persistence of these free radicals is a necessary, but not a sufficient, condition for further polymerisation, for instance, at elevated temperatures [84–86].

DMTA and DETA

DMTA and DETA were used to investigate the formation of network in dental resin formulations [87].

Development of Mechanical Properties;;

Surface Hardness

The hardness of the top surface of a VLC composite resin specimen is observed to increase with time at ambient temperatures after the cessation of light irradiation, although there has been variation in the reported time scale [88–90]. The surface hardness changes should at least partially reflect changes in the bulk properties. An empirical mathematical model was proposed for this effect by Johnson et al. [91] based on non-linear regression. This incorporates exponential terms of the form derived previously, but involves two time constants.

Bulk Elastic and Visco-Elastic Compliance

The time dependence of development of Young's modulus in flexure was reported [92], and this followed a similar pattern to that of shrinkage and hardness. Similar changes in visco-elastic properties, such as static creep and creep recovery [93], are apparent following cure initiation as the network develops.

General Polymerisation Mechanism for Light-Activated Monomers

The principal chain-reaction steps involved subsequent to photo-activation of free radicals (A^*) are as follows, with the associated rate constants [$k_{...}$]:

Initiation [k_i]	A^*	+	M	6	AM
Propagation [k_p]	$M_n^{\bullet}$	+	M	6	$M_{n+1}^{\bullet}$
Termination [k_t]	$M_n^{\bullet}$	+	$M_m^{'}$	6	$M_{(n+m)}$
Inhibition/retardation [k_x]	$M_n^{\bullet}$	+	X	6	$M_nX^{\bullet}$ (inactive)
	$R^{\bullet}$	+	X	6	$RX^{\bullet}$ (inactive)

A, M and X denote the photo-reducer (usually an amine), the monomer and the inhibitor, while R and M_n are the initiator and polymer radicals. In the presence of certain chemicals, chain transfer is a further mechanistic possibility.

An active centre is created when a free radical attacks the π-bond of a molecule of monomer. Propagation involves growth of the polymer chain by rapid sequential addition of monomer to the active centre. With vinyl chain polymerisation (e.g. methyl methacrylate or methacrylate end groups) there is head to tail or head to head; the former predominates because attack at the methylene [CH_2=] carbon is less sterically hindered and yields a product free radical that is stable because of the effects of the adjacent side chain. The time required for each monomer addition is typically a millisecond.

Steady-State Hypotheses

Simplifying assumptions are commonly made in the development of equations in chemical kinetics; these concern either an assumed or a demonstrable balance in rate processes between the production and destruction of intermediate molecular species. In the present case, three such assumptions are made, concerning:

1. Excited states of CQ (singlet and triplet). Radiation in the visible region (400–550 nm, where max=470 nm) promotes an electron in one of the two carbonyl groups of CQ to a short-lived, excite state. The half-life is approximately 0.05 ms for the CQ triplet [57].
2. Initiator radicals. The CQ/amine photoinitiator system for generating radicals is widely used for the polymerisation of dental restorative materials.
3. Polymer chain radicals. If the light irradiance is very high, then the system(s) may not be in balance, and so the steady-state assumptions may not hold.

Polymerisation Kinetics of Light-Activated Resin Composites

The following analytical equations may be developed for photo-polymerisation kinetics for linear-chain systems.

The rate of production of primary free radicals from the photo-sensitiser (R_r) can be formally expressed by:

$$R_r = 2\phi I_a$$

where I_a is the light intensity absorbed by the photo-sensitiser across a thickness element δd, at depth d in the medium (as calculated above) and φ is the quantum yield for initiation [94, 95]. The factor 2 is strictly optional and is usually used when two radicals are generated for each photo-sensitiser molecule. As already noted, however, of the two, radicals generated according to the photo-activation scheme that derived from the amine has the greater efficiency in initiation.

A detailed kinetic analysis of the activation steps has been made by Cook [96]. This can be re-expressed via the following expression for R_r which amounts to a calculation of the quantum yield in terms of underlying mechanistic quantities:

$$R_r = \beta\, k_a\, [A]\, [Q^*{}_T]$$

where β is the fraction of exciplex "molecules" forming free radicals, and k_a is the rate constant for exciplex formation from bimolecular reaction between amine and triplet-CQ.

The lifetimes of excited singlet states are normally very short, so the concentration of $Q^*{}_S$ should be low, also the concentration of the triplet $Q^*{}_T$ should be low and unchanging (the "steady-state" assumption); thus:

$$d[Q^*{}_S]/dt = d[Q^*{}_T]/dt = 0,$$

and hence it can be shown that (where $k' = k_1 + k_2$):

$$Q^*{}_T = k_2\, \varepsilon_Q\, [Q]\, I / \{k'.k_3 + k'.k_a\, [A]\}$$

where, as above, I is the light irradiance at depth d in the material. Also, the other quantities are defined above and/or in the reaction scheme.

Some consequences of practical importance follow from this analysis: there are limiting cases for the kinetic equations, corresponding to high or low amine concentrations:

At high [A], R_r is *in*dependent of [A].
At low [A], R_r is dependent on [A].

Since most resin composites are viscous and form a gel structure at low degrees of conversion (ca. 15%), it can be assumed that the photo-sensitiser and resultant free radicals do not rapidly diffuse [97]; thus, if the further steady-state assumption is made that the rates of production and consumption of initiator radicals rapidly become equal, then R_r is equal to the rate of initiation (R_i). This assumption will require a concentration of photo-reducer [A] to be present that matches that of the photo-initiator [Q].

Rate of Polymerisation

The rate of monomer disappearance, which is synonymous with the rate of polymerisation, is given by the sum of the rates of initiation and propagation, R_i and R_p, since both steps consume monomer; however, the former term (R_i) is relatively insignificant and can be neglected, so

$$-\frac{d[M]}{dt} = R_p = k_p[M^*][M]$$

where [M] is the monomer concentration and [M] is the total concentration of all chain radicals of size M_1 and larger.

Normal Termination Model

If a steady-state assumption is again made that the concentration of polymer radicals rapidly attains a constant value, then this is equivalent to saying that the rates of initiation and normal termination are equal, and hence:

$$R_i = 2k_t[M^*]^2$$

Rearrangement and substitution into the preceding equation yields:

$$R_p = k_p[M]\left\{\frac{R_i}{2k_t}\right\}^{0.5}$$

The first expression for R_r may be substituted for R_i in this equation to give

$$R_p = -\frac{d[M]}{dt} = k_p[M]\left\{\frac{\phi I_a}{k_t}\right\}^{0.5}$$

This gives us the important result that the rate of polymerisation is proportional to the square root of the absorbed light irradiance, and hence proportional to the square root of the photo-initiator concentration.

This rate equation may be integrated with respect to time (t) from commencement of irradiation to give an expression for the *degree of conversion* (DC):

$$DC = \int_0^t R_p dt = \int_0^t -\frac{d[M]}{dt} dt$$

$$DC = \left(\frac{M_0 - M}{M_0}\right) = 1 - e^{-k_p k_t^{-0.5}(\phi I_\alpha{}^{0.5}.t)}$$

M_0 is the initial concentration of methacrylate groups and M is the concentration at time (t). This equation, in conjunction with preceding expressions relating absorbed light (I_a) to incident light intensity, predicts that at constant DC the maximum value for depth of cure (d_{max}) is directly related to both *log* I_0 and *log* (irradiation time) with slopes of 1/a and 2/a [98]. These last two polymerisation-rate expressions, in differential and integral form, are related further to polymerisation shrinkage kinetics and to the development of surface hardness and bulk mechanical properties [99, 100]. The preceding analysis may be extended to predict that the number-average molecular mass of polymer chains, in the case of linear polymerisation (e.g. of methyl methacrylate), is inversely proportional to the square root of photo-initiator concentration. Qualitatively, this is understood in terms of many initiator centres resulting in relatively short chains, and vice versa, because of a finite pool of monomer molecules.

Auto-Acceleration

There is often a sharp increase in R_p as the conversion of monomer increases. This phenomenon is known as auto-acceleration or the Trommsdorf-Norrish effect or the gel effect. Auto-acceleration arises as a consequence of the increase in viscosity and temperature of the reaction medium caused by the formation of polymer molecules which leads to a rapid decrease in the termination rate constant k_t.

The contrast between linear and cross-linking reactions is extensively reviewed by Andrzejewska [101]. Figure 6.6 shows the contrast in kinetic profile (rate of polymerisation vs time) for these two situations. It is apparent that the polymerisation rate in crosslinking systems shows auto-acceleration followed by auto-deceleration.

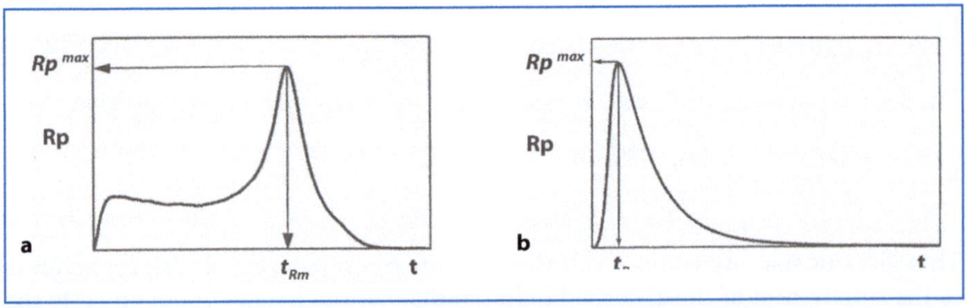

Fig. 6.6 a, b. Typical shape of kinetic curve of polymerisation rate as a function of irradiation time for the polymerisation of **a** monomethacrylate monomer and **b** dimethacrylate

Definitions of Polymerisation Shrinkage Phenomena

Polymerisation Shrinkage Strain: How Much? How Fast? What Direction?

The polymerisation of dental composite resins is inevitably accompanied by shrinkage. Existing types of photo-curable resins and composites, especially those based on acrylates and methacrylates, exhibit polymerisation shrinkage of monomers during the setting process. Polymerisation shrinkage strain of resin composites, particularly shrinkage in a direction normal to the interface of the material with dental tissues, is of critical importance [102]. Plastic flow may occur during the pre-gelation phase such that internal stresses within the material undergo stress relaxation [103]. Beyond the gel point, however, stress development occurs. Its magnitude, relative to the strain, depends on the elastic (or visco-elastic) moduli, which are also increasing functions of time [92]. Polymerisation stresses in a bonded structure may cause adhesive or cohesive failure and interfacial gap formation or, if adhesion is maintained, deformation of residual tooth structure may occur.

Shrinkage is a vector quantity and composite shrinkage patterns are often anisotropic, especially when the material is placed in an open cavity. The adverse effects of polymerisation shrinkage stress on the bond between restorative materials and hard tissues have been extensively described in the dental literature [13, 17, 104].

Following the onset of cure, the post-gelation rigid shrinkage is the factor of clinical significance. Flow may compensate for the effects of shrinkage during the pre-gelation phase; however, VLC resin composites reach the gel point rapidly, typically at 15% conversion. The present generation of flowable composites undergo a free volumetric shrinkage of 4–9% [105]. For condensable composites volumetric shrinkage is in the range 2.0–6.0%, with most values near 3.5% [6]. Sixty-five to 75% of this shrinkage occurs within the first 10 min of placement, irrespective of curing mode [106].

Polymerisation shrinkage can be influenced by various factors. Increasing the volume of inert material, be it inorganic or organic filler, *may* reduce the overall shrinkage of composites, simply because less monomer is present to react [107]; however, towards the upper limit of filler fraction there is increased viscosity that results in a clay-like paste. Then monomers are added as diluents to reduce resin. Also, high filler loading results in a high degree of stiffness, which can lead to high shrinkage stress; hence, increases in volume fraction of filler do not invariably produce a substantial reduction in shrinkage [72].

The magnitude of polymerisation shrinkage is also dependent on the extent of the reaction, and its ability to flow. Another factor is the monomer size. The larger a molecule is, the less the polymerisation shrinkage for a given volume [108, 109].

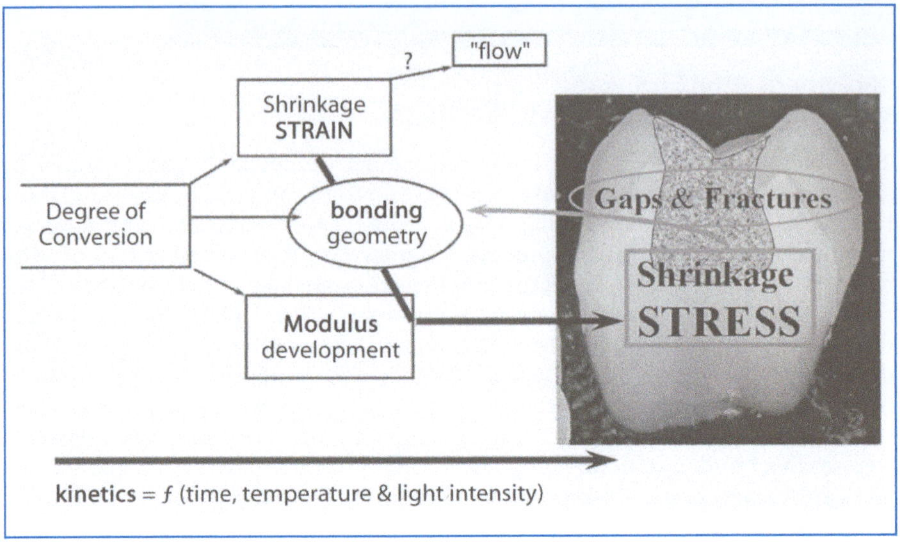

Fig. 6.7. Diagrammatic relationships of polymerisation shrinkage phenomena

Shrinkage Stress

Polymerisation shrinkage stress is not only a function of the composite's volumetric shrinkage strain, but it is also determined by its visco-elastic behaviour, which is usually described in terms of elastic modulus development and flow capacity. Generally, the higher the volumetric shrinkage and/or the faster the material acquires elastic properties after the beginning of polymerisation, the higher the stresses will be. On the other hand, at early stages of polymerisation, before the onset of gelation (known as "gel point"), crosslinking density is relatively low and the polymeric chains may assume new positions (flow), permitting stress relaxation.

The inter-relationships between stress and strain are shown in Fig. 6.7.

Generation of Stresses in Different Cavity Configurations (C-Factor)

C-factor is the ratio of the bonded to unbonded surface area of the specimen:

C = total bonded area/total unbonded area

Feilzer et al. showed the role of cavity configuration (C-factor) on the development of polymerisation stresses with in a resin composite [110]. They described an in vitro model in which restorations, with C-factor <1, are the only ones likely to survive polymerisation shrinkage stresses; thus, early bond strengths are crucial since they are responsible for preserving the adhesive interface during development of stress from polymerisation. Therefore, the magnitude of the shrinkage stress is dependent on material properties [111], on the cavity configuration

(C-factor) [112] and on the amount of compliance of the surrounding structures [7, 113].

Several studies reported reductions of bond strength values under high C-factor cavities [114–116].

Generally, the less the free, unbonded area there is in a cavity, the less will be the ability of resin to flow, and therefore the greater will be the shrinkage stress at the bonded surfaces.

If a small fraction of the bond is broken during polymerisation shrinkage of the resins, the retention of the resin composite may not be significantly affected; however, the seal of the restoration is compromised and may lead to undesirable clinical consequences. This hypothesis may also explain the lack of a good correlation between bond strength and marginal leakage data [117, 118]. To achieve good dentin bonding, the forces of polymerisation shrinkage must be minimised and dentin bond strengths must be maximised.

Measurement of Shrinkage Strain

For more than a decade, several techniques have been developed and utilised for measurement of shrinkage strain. Composite shrinkage has been determined from dilatometric [119], linometer [120] and "bonded-disk" methods (Fig. 6.8) [100] where the shrinkage may occur in one dimension, normal to the specimen surface. Other methods include laser interferometry [121] and differential variable transducer [122].

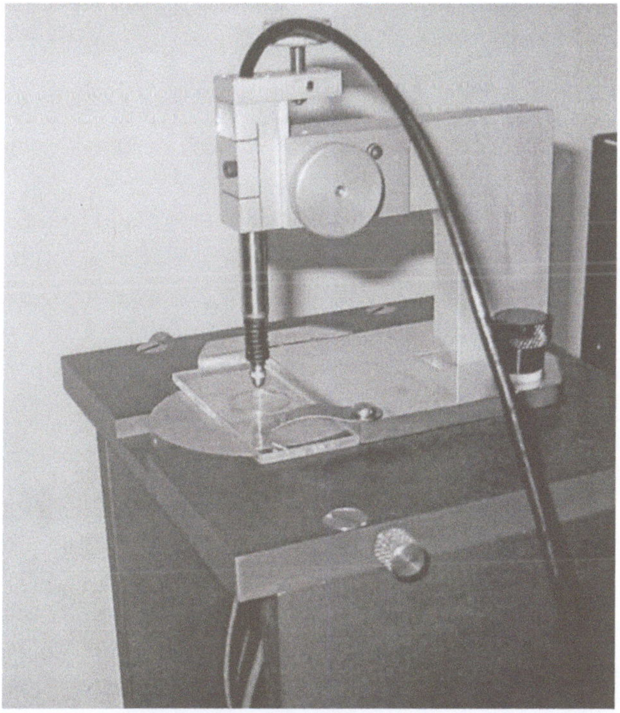

Fig. 6.8. Bonded-disk apparatus for shrinkage-strain measurement

Kinetics of Shrinkage Strain

The theory of polymerisation kinetics, discussed above, predicts an exponential growth curve for shrinkage vs time, provided that (a) there is a steady-state concentration of polymer radicals, with radicals disappearing by normal termination, and (b) the shrinkage kinetics keep in step with the crosslinking polymerisation. The time constant (τ) is then inversely proportional to the square root of the irradiance of light (I_a), of appropriate wavelength, absorbed by the photosensitiser.

Once initiated, the initial rigid polymerisation shrinkage of VLC resin composites proceeds rapidly, in a near-linear manner with time. For most materials, however, the normalised overall decay in free volume (V), i.e., shrinkage, was approximately represented by the Kohlrausch-Williams-Watts (KWW) stretched-exponential relaxation function, [123, 124]:

$$\Delta V/V_0 = 1 - e^{-(t/\tau)^\beta}$$

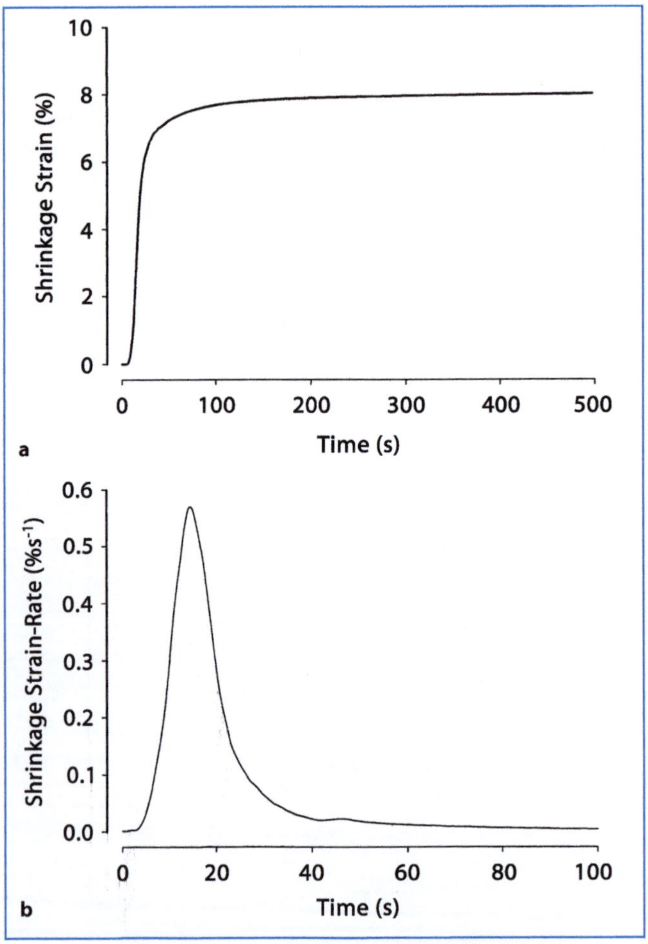

Fig. 6.9 a, b. Representative shrinkage-strain data for a dimethacrylate monomer system, from the bonded-disk method. **a** Strain vs time; **b** strain rate vs time

where $0<\beta\leq 1$, typical values being 0.3–0.6. This is particularly appropriate to the situation following the initial linear shrinkage. The glassy state is swiftly generated by photo-polymerisation and the KWW function characterises the time dependence of segmental motion in the glassy state as a fractal-time stochastic process [123], which is the governing factor for the self-limiting processes of bulk polymerisation and free-volume shrinkage. Representative shrinkage-strain and strain-rate data, from the bonded-disk method, are shown in Fig. 6.9.

Relationship Between *DC* and Shrinkage Strain

Volumetric shrinkage is directly related to the *degree of conversion* of composites [3, 4]. Higher degrees of conversion are usually associated with improved mechanical properties; therefore, there is a myth that high degrees of conversion would improve the performance of composite restorations over time. However, higher degrees of conversion will also lead to higher contraction stresses. It was shown that the stress-development rate increases at higher conversion levels [125]. Optimum *DC* and minimal polymerisation shrinkage are generally antagonistic goals.

Theoretical Relationship Between Conversion and Shrinkage Strain

In the polymer science literature it is widely accepted that the dominant cause of shrinkage strain in mono-methacrylates arises from conversion of C=C double bonds, where for each monomer segment of the chain the larger van der Waals inter-molecular spacing is replaced by the smaller intra-molecular covalent bond [126, 127]. This results in density changes on proceeding from monomer to polymer [128]; thus, an exact semi-empirical relationship can be derived.

Experimentally, the volume change per mole of methacrylate groups (C=C) in methylmethacrylate (MMA) is:

$$DV_{C=C} = 22.5\ \text{cm}^3/\text{mole}\ [\text{or}\ 10^{-6}\ \text{m}^3/\text{mole}]$$

[126, 129] when MMA is polymerised. The molar volume of MMA is:

$$\frac{M_m}{\rho_m} = \frac{100.12}{0.94} = 106.51\text{cm}^3.$$

Hence, the volumetric shrinkage strain of MMA is $\frac{22.5}{106.5} \times 110 = 21.12\,\%$.

where

M_m is the molecular weight and ϱ_m is the density.

The values for density and molecular weight were obtained from the Polymer Handbook [130]. In the more general case of multi-methacrylates, where f is the functionality of the monomer, the number of functional groups present in volume (V) is:

$$\left[f \times \frac{V \cdot \rho_m}{M_m}\right]$$

The number of functional groups reacted in volume (V) is:

$$DC \times \left[f \times \frac{V \cdot \rho_m}{M_m}\right]$$

where DC is the fractional *degree of conversion*.

The percentage relative change in volume (volumetric shrinkage strain) is:

$$\frac{\Delta V}{V}(\%) = 22.5 \times DC \times f \times \frac{V \cdot \rho_m}{M_m} \times 100 \qquad (1)$$

For a mixture of monomers of any functionality:

$$\frac{\Delta V}{V}(\%) = 22.5 \times DC_{mix} \cdot \frac{\sum_i (f_i \cdot \chi_i)}{\sum_i (M_{mi} \cdot \chi_i)} \cdot \rho_{mix} \cdot 100 \qquad (2)$$

For example, with two monomers, one monofunctional and one difunctional

$$\frac{\Delta V}{V}(\%) = 22.5 \times DC_{mix} \cdot \left[\frac{2.\chi_1 + \chi_2}{M_{m1} \cdot \chi_1 + M_{m2} \cdot \chi_2}\right] \cdot \rho_{mix} \cdot 100 \qquad (3)$$

Equations (1)–(3) embody the expectation that the volumetric shrinkage strain will be directly proportional to the DC of the monomer systems; hence, if the DC diminishes for any reason, the shrinkage strain should also be observed to decrease [131].

Experimental Correlations between *DC* and Shrinkage-Strain Magnitudes

The DC and shrinkage-strain values of two resin composites (Z100 and TRC) were measured. The irradiance used was varied systematically, but each set of samples prepared for DC and shrinkage-strain experiments were exposed to the same light irradiance; therefore, a meaningful correlation between the two methods was established. Significant reductions in light intensity by a factor of ca. 3.8 only reduced DC by a factor of 1.3 for TCR and 1.6 for Z100 as measured by FTIR [3].

The results obtained from the shrinkage-strain measurements showed a significant decrease in shrinkage strain when light intensity was decreased. This decrease in shrinkage, if sustained, could lead to better marginal adaptation.

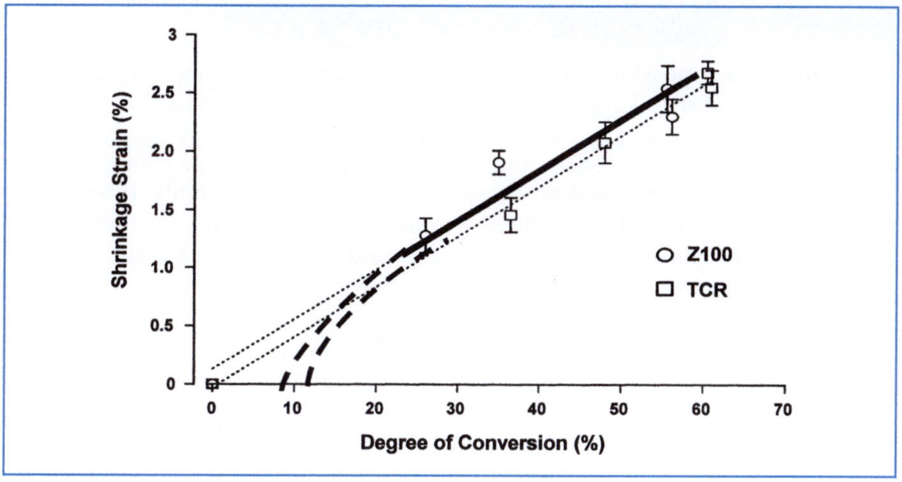

Fig. 6.10. Relationships between *degree of conversion* and shrinkage strain for two resin composites: Tetric Ceram (*TRC*) and Z100. The points on each graph were for increasing light-irradiance levels applied to the composites, for both DC and shrinkage measurements, resulting in progressively greater monomer conversion

The correlation shown in Fig. 6.10 is restricted to the range 26–61% *DC*. Extrapolation to lower *DC* values should be done with care. It is possible, as indicated by the dashed lines, that the plot could become curvilinear, so that it would express the possibility of zero shrinkage despite a finite *DC* (ca. 10%); hence, a close relationship between *DC* and shrinkage strain, with antagonistic clinical implications, was confirmed.

Network Variables Beyond *Degree of Conversion*

Although *degree of conversion* is the most important parameter for characterising a dental composite network, it is not the only possible structural factor of interest. Different irradiation modes may result in the same *DC* but differing network structures. Exposure to suitable solvents, followed by surface hardness measurements, has been explored as a means of investigation [132].

Measurement of Shrinkage-Stress Kinetics

Several methods now exist for measurement of the final shrinkage-stress magnitude generated by a composite in a defined host environment. Methods that determine the kinetic development of shrinkage stress with time are particularly useful. One such method, using the Bioman instrument, incorporates a cantilever load-cell geometry [133, 134].

Scientific Management of Shrinkage Phenomena

There are several possible approaches to producing resin-composite materials that have reduced shrinkage strain and/or reduced shrinkage stress.

1. Adjustments to existing resin chemistry. Various modified dimethacrylate monomer mixtures are being investigated to reduce shrinkage phenomena.
2. Adjustments to dispersed-phase filler technology. The highly filler-loaded materials generally exhibit reduced shrinkage strain; however, the high moduli of these materials do not generally lead to reduced shrinkage stress.
3. The quest for new resin chemistry.

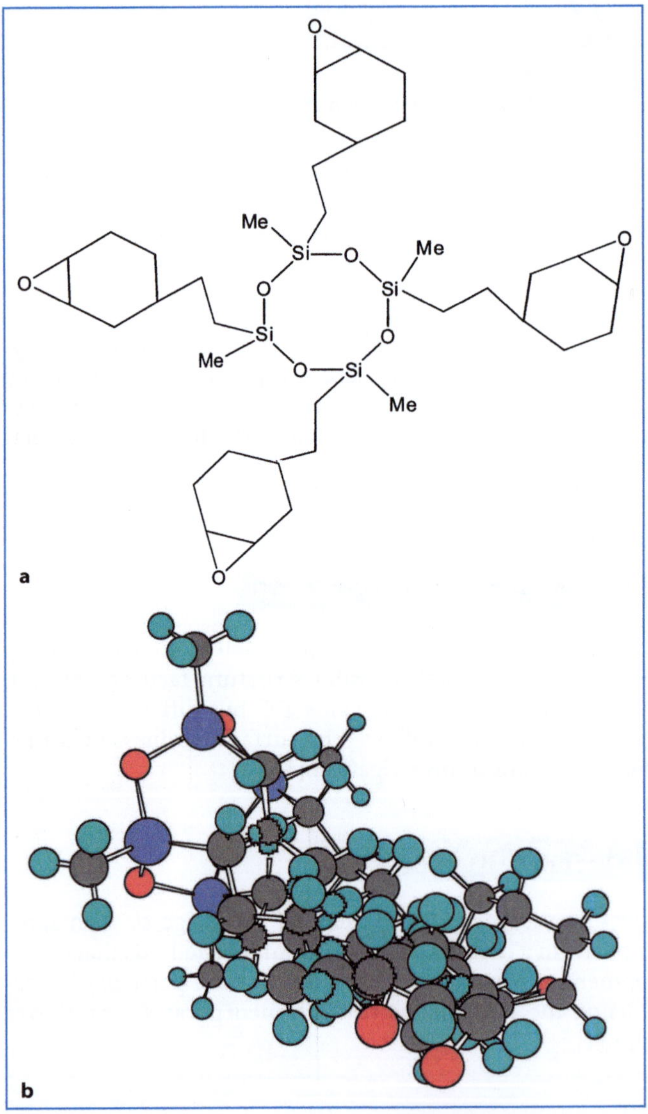

Fig. 6.11 a, b. Chemical structures of silorane monomer, in **a** 2D and **b** 3D stick-and-ball model. *Purple* Si; *red* O; *black* C; *green* H

Progress towards elimination or reduction of polymerisation shrinkage by synthesis of monomers that expand upon polymerisation has been reported by Thompson et al. [135] and Stansbury [14]. New developments have arisen using epoxide and silorane chemistry (Fig. 6.11).

Conclusion

The polymerisation of resins is invariably accompanied by the volumetric shrinkage of the cured material compared with the unset state. Shrinkage is associated with the polymerisation reaction in a complex way. The reduction in shrinkage strain could be attributed to reduced network connectivity, or to an increased propensity for flow of the materials. Throughout the entire polymerisation process, plastic deformation or flow of the composite resin may occur to a limited extent, until vitrification occurs. Reduced light irradiance may result in a storage modulus development at a slow enough rate to allow for flow and dissipation of stress, while maintaining a sufficient bond to tooth structure. As the setting process proceeds, shrinkage and flow decrease gradually because storage modulus increases. Under high light irradiance, composite resins restrain this stress relief much more by not allowing enough flow to reduce internal stress. Restriction of the flow capacity by the configuration of the restoration also enhances the shrinkage stress; hence, optimal rheological effects would enhance marginal adaptation. These beneficial effects of flow are being utilised when decreased light intensity is employed. The practice of "soft-start" polymerisation utilises the foregoing theory.

With regard to optimal light-curing intensities for clinical purposes, the minimum amount of irradiation for direct curing and indirect curing through enamel or dentine is still unknown. High curing intensities may not be essential. Low intensities will slow the reaction. As the rate of conversion determines the rate of shrinkage, stress development and the ultimate stress level, any retardation of the reaction will contribute to slowing down the shrinkage stress development and possibly its ultimate value. This will be primarily achieved by the extended time period for some viscous flow, which may compensate for the developing stresses.

References

1. Watts DC, Al Hindi A. Intrinsic "soft-start" polymerisation shrinkage-kinetics in an acrylate-based resin-composite. Dent Mater 1999; 15:39–45
2. Versluis A, Douglas WH, Cross M, Sakaguchi RL. Does an incremental filling technique reduce polymerization shrinkage stresses? J Dent Res 1996; 75:871–878
3. Silikas N, Eliades G, Watts DC. Light intensity effects on resin-composite degree of conversion and shrinkage strain. Dent Mater 2000; 16:292–296
4. Sakaguchi R, Berge H. Reduced light energy density decreases post-gel contraction while maintaining degree of conversion in composites. J Dent 1998; 26:695–700
5. Pananakis D, Watts DC. Incorporation of the heating effect of the light source in a non-isothermal model of a visible-light-cured resin composite. J Mater Sci 2000; 35:4589–4600
6. Labella R, Lambrechts P, Van Meerbeek B, Vanherle G. Polymerisation shrinkage and elasticity of flowable composites and filled adhesives. Dent Mater 1999; 15:128–137

7. Davidson CL, Feilzer AJ. Polymerisation shrinkage and polymerisation shrinkage stress in polymer-based restoratives. J Dent 1997; 25:435–440
8. Kinomoto Y, Torii M, Takeshige F, Ebisu S. Comparison of polymerization contraction stresses between self- and light-curing composites. J Dent Res 1999; 27:383–389
9. Hegdahl T, Gjerdet NR. Contraction stresses of composite resin filling materials. Acta Odont Scand 1977; 35:191–195
10. Condon JR, Ferracane JL. Reduction of composite contraction stress through non-bonded microfiller particles. Dent Mater 1998; 14:256–260
11. Carvalho RM, Pereira JC, Yoshiyama M, Pashley DH. A review of polymerisation contraction: the influence of stress development versus stress relief. Oper Dent 1996; 21:17–24
12. Bouchlicher MR, Vargas MA, Boyer DB. Effect of composite type, light intensity, configuration factor and laser polymerisation on polymerisation contraction forces. Am J Dent 1997; 10:88–96
13. Eick JD, Welch FW. Polymerisation shrinkage of posterior composite resins and its possible influence on postoperative sensitivity. Quintessence Int 1986; 17:103–111
14. Stansbury JW. Cyclopolymerisable monomers for use in dental resin composites. J Dent Res 1990; 69:844–848
15. Sakaguchi RL, Ferracane JL. Stress transfer from polymerization shrinkage of a chemical-cured composite bonded to a pre-cast composite substrate. Dent Mater 1998; 14:106–111
16. Feilzer AJ, Dooren LH, de Gee AJ, Davidson CL. Influence of light intensity on polymerization shrinkage and integrity of restoration–cavity interface. Eur J Oral Sci 1995; 103:322–326
17. Sakaguchi R, Brust E, Cross M, DeLong R, Douglas W. Independent movement of cusps during occlusal loading. Dent Mater 1991; 7:186–190
18. Tantbirojn D, Versluis A, Pintado M, DeLong R, Douglas W. Tooth deformation patterns in molars after composite restoration. Dent Mater 2004; 20:535–542
19. Morin DL, Douglas WH, Cross M. Biophysical stress analysis of restored teeth: experimental strain measurement. Dent Mater 1988; 4:41–48
20. Opdam N, Roeters F, Feilzer A, Verdonschot E. Marginal integrity and postoperative sensitivity in class 2 resin composite restorations in vivo. J Dent 1998; 26:555–562
21. Lopes G, Baratieri L, Monteiro SJ, Vieira L. Effect of posterior resin composite placement technique on the resin–dentin interface formed in vivo. Quintessence Int 2004; 35:156–161
22. Althof O, Hartung M. Advances in light curing. Am J Dent 2000; 13:77D–81D
23. Hofmann N, Hugo B, Schubert K, Klaiber B. Comparison between a plasma arc light source and conventional halogen curing units regarding flexural strength, modulus, and hardness of photoactivated resin composites. Clin Oral Investig 2000; 4:140–147
24. Peutzfeldt A, Sahafi A, Asmussen E. Characterization of resin composites polymerized with plasma arc curing units. Dent Mater 2000; 16:330–336
25. Blankenau R, Erickson R, Rueggeberg F. New light curing options for composite resin restorations. Compend Contin Educ Dent 1999; 20:122–125
26. Bennett A, Watts D. Performance of two blue light-emitting-diode dental light curing units with distance and irradiation time. Dent Mater 2004; 20:72–79
27. Smith F. Optics and photonics, an introduction. Wiley, New York, 2000
28. Mills RW. Blue light emitting diodes: another method of light curing? Br Dent J 1995; 178:169
29. Jandt K, Blackwell G, Ashworth S. Depth of cure and compressive strength of dental composite cured with blue light emitting diodes (LEDs). Dent Mater 2000; 16:41–44
30. Yap A, Soh M, Siow K. Post-gel shrinkage with pulse activation and soft-start polymerization. Oper Dent 2002; 27:81–87
31. Soh M, Yap A. Influence of curing modes on crosslink density in polymer structures. J Dent 2004; 32:321–326
32. Hofmann N, Denner W, Hugo B, Klaiber B. The influence of plasma arc vs halogen standard or soft-start irradiation on polymerization shrinkage kinetics of polymer matrix composites. J Dent 2003; 31:383–393
33. Hofmann N, Markert T, Hugo B, Klaiber B. Effect of high intensity vs soft-start halogen irradiation on light-cured resin-based composites. Part I. Temperature rise and polymerization shrinkage. Am J Dent 2003; 16:421–430

34. Hofmann N, Markert T, Hugo B, Klaiber B. Effect of high intensity vs soft-start halogen irradiation on light-cured resin-based composites. Part II. Hardness and solubility. Am J Dent 2004; 17:38–42
35. Bouschlicher M, Rueggeberg F. Effect of ramped light intensity on polymerization force and conversion in a photoactivated composite. J Esthet Dent 2000; 12:328–339
36. De Lange C, Bausch J, Davidson C. The curing pattern of photo-initiated dental composites. J Oral Rehab 1980; 7:369–377
37. Watts D, Amer O, Combe E. Characteristics of visible light-cured composite systems. Br Dent J 1984; 156:209–215
38. Ruyter IF. Methacrylate-based polymeric dental materials: conversion and related properties. Summary and review. Acta Odontol Scand 1982; 40:359–376
39. Rueggeberg F, Craig R. Correlation of parameters used to estimate monomer conversion in a light-cured composite. J Dent Res 1988; 67:932–937
40. Ferracane J. Correlation between hardness and degree of conversion during the setting reaction of unfilled dental restorative resins. Dent Mater 1985; 1:11–14
41. DeWald J, Ferracane J. A comparison of four modes of evaluating depth of cure of light-activated composites. J Dent Res 1987; 66:727–730
42. Cook WD, Standish P. Cure of resin-based restorative materials. II. White light photo-polymerised resins. Aust Dent J 1983; 28:307–311
43. Miyagawa Y, Powers J. Prediction of color of an esthetic restorative material. J Dent Res 1983; 62:581
44. Van Krevelen D. Properties of polymers. Elsevier, Amsterdam, 1976
45. Kubelka P, Munk F. A contribution to the optics of pigments. Z Technol Phys 1931; 12:593
46. Miyagawa Y, Powers J, O'Brian W. Optical properties of direct restorative materials. J Dent Res 1981; 60:890
47. Cook W, McAree D. Optical properties of esthetic restorative materials and natural dentition. J Biomed Mater Res 1985; 19:469
48. Taira M, Yamaki M. Studies on optical properties of a visible-light-cured dental composite resin by diffuse reflectance measurements. J Mater Sci Lett 1995; 14:198
49. Wozniak W, Siew E, Lim J, McGill S, Sabri Z, Moser J. Color mixing in dental porcelain. Dent Mater 1993; 9:229
50. Lee Y, Powers J. Color and optical properties of resin-based composites for bleached teeth after polymerization and accelerated aging. Am J Dent 2001; 14:349–354
51. McCabe J, Carrick T. Output from visible-light activation units and depth of cure of light-activated composites. J Dent Res 1989; 68:1534–1539
52. Suzuki H, Taira M, Wakasa K, Yamaki M. Refractive-index-adjustable fillers for visible-light-cured dental resin composites: preparation of TiO_2–SiO_2 glass powder by the sol-gel process. J Dent Res 1991; 70:883
53. Moad G, Chiefari J, Mayadunne R et al. Initiating free radical polymerization. Macromol Sympos 2002; 182:65–80
54. Dart E, Nemcek J. British Patent 1975:1 408 265
55. Taira M, Urabe H, Hirose T, Wakasa K, Yamaki M. Analysis of photo initiators in visible light-cured dental composite resins. J Dent Res 1988; 67:24–28
56. Tsai L, Charney E. The triplet states of a-Dicarbonyls. J Phys Chem 1969; 73:2462–2463
57. Stansbury J. Curing dental resins and composites by photopolymerization. J Esthet Dent 2000; 12:300–308
58. Peutzfeldt A, Asmussen E. Effect of propanal and diacetyl on quantity of remaining double bonds of chemically cured BisGMA/TEGDMA resins. Eur J Oral Sci 1996; 104:309–312
59. Peutzfeldt A, Asmussen E. In vitro wear, hardness, and conversion of diacetyl-containing and propanal-containing resin materials. Dent Mater 1996; 12:103–108
60. Chae K-H, Sun G-J. Phenylpropanedione; a new visible light photosensitizer for dental composite resin with higher efficiency than camphorquinone. Bull Korean Chem Soc 1998; 19:152–154
61. Sun G, Chae K. Properties of 2,3-butanedione and 1-phenyl-1,2-propanedione as new photosensitizers for visible light cured dental resin composites. Polymer 2000; 41:6205–6212

62. Park Y-J, Chaec K-H, Rawlsa HR. Development of a new photoinitiation system for dental light-cure composite resins. Dent Mater 1999; 15:120–127
63. Ferracane J, Greener E. Fourier transform infrared analysis of degree of polymerization in unfilled resins: methods comparison. J Dent Res 1984; 63:1093–1095
64. Ferracane JL, Greener EH. The effect of resin formulation on the degree of conversion and mechanical properties of dental restorative resins. J Biomed Mater Res 1986; 20:121–131
65. Eliades GG, Vougiouklakis GJ, Caputo AA. Degree of double bond conversion in light-cured composites. Dent Mater 1987; 3:19–25
66. Ruyter I, Oysaed H. Analysis and characterization of dental polymers. Crit Rev Biocompat 1988; 4:247–279
67. Cox C, Keall C, Keall H, Ostro E, Bergenholtz G. Biocompatibility of surface-sealed dental materials against exposed pulps. J Prosth Dent 1987; 57:1–8
68. Vankerckhoven H, Lambrechts P, Van Beylen M, Vanherle G. Unreacted methacrylate groups on the surfaces of composite resins. J Dent Res 1982; 61:791–795
69. Ruyter IE, Svendsen S. Remaining methacrylate groups in composite restorative materials. Acta Odontol Scand 1978; 36:75–82
70. Asmussen E. Factors affecting the quantity of remaining double bonds in restorative resin polymers. Scand Dent Res 1982; 90:490–496
71. Maffezzoli A, Terzi R. Thermal analysis of visible-light-activated dental composites. Thermochim Acta 1995; 269/270:319–335
72. Ferracane JL. In vitro evaluation of resin composites. Structure-property relationships. Development of assessment criteria. Trans Acad Dent Mater 1989; 2:6–35
73. Scherzer T. Real-time FTIR-ATR spectroscopy of photopolymerization reactions. Macromol Sympos 2002; 184:79–97
74. Oréfice R, Disacciati J, Neves A, Mansur H, Jansen W. In situ evaluation of the polymerization kinetics and corresponding evolution of the mechanical properties of dental composites. Polymer Testing 2003; 22:77–81
75. Stansbury J, Dickens S. Determination of double bond conversion in dental resins by near infrared spectroscopy. Dent Mater 2001; 17:71–79
76. Louden J, Roberts T. Cure profiles of light-cured dental composites by Raman spectroscopy. J Ram Spec 1983; 14:365–366
77. Pianelli C, Devaux J, Bebelman S, Leloup G. The micro-raman spectroscopy, a useful tool to determine the degree of conversion of light-activated composite resins. J Biomed Mater Res (Appl Biomater) 1999; 48:675–681
78. Emami N, Soderholm K-JM, Berglund L. Effect of light power density variations on bulk curing properties of dental composites. J Dent 2003; 31:189–196
79. Tsuda H, Arends J. Raman spectroscopy in dental research: a short review of recent studies. Adv Dent Res 1997; 11:539–547
80. Miyazaki M, Onose H, Moore B. Analysis of the dentin–resin interface by use of laser Raman spectroscopy. Dent Mater 2002; 18:576–580
81. Heatley F, Pratsitsilp Y, McHugh N, Watts D, Devlin H. Determination of extent of reaction in dimethacrylate-based dental composites using solid-state 13 C m.a.s. n.m.r. spectroscopy and comparison with FTi.r. spectroscopy. Polymer 1995; 36:1859–1867
82. Pereira S, Nunes T, Kalachandra S. Low viscosity dimethacrylate comonomer compositions [Bis-GMA and CH3Bis-GMA] for novel dental composites; analysis of the network by stray-field MRI, solid-state NMR and DSC & FTIR. Biomaterials 2002; 23:3799–3806
83. Teshima W, Nomura Y, Tanaka N, Urabe H, Okazaki M, Nahara Y. ESR study of camphorquinone/amine photoinitiator systems using blue light-emitting diodes. Biomaterials 2003; 24:2097–2103
84. Anseth KS, Anderson KJ, Bowman CN. Radical concentrations, environments, and reactivities during crosslinking polymerizations. Macromol Chem Phys 1996; 197:833–848
85. Mizuta Y, Morishita N, Kuwata K. Propagating radicals in photo-initiated polymerization as detected by time-resolved CW- and FT-ESR spectroscopy. Chem Lett 1999:311–312

86. Selli E, Oliva C, Galbiati M, Bellobono I. EPR investigation of radical formation and decay in photopolymerization of difunctional monomers. J Chem Soc Perkin Trans 1992; 2:1391–1395
87. Jancar J, Wang W, Benedetto A di. On the heterogeneous structure of thermally cured bis-GMA/TEGDMA resins. J Mater Sci Mater Med 2000; 11:675–682
88. Leung RL, Fan PL, Jonston WM. Post-irradiation polymerization of visible light-activated composite resin. J Dent Res 1983; 62:363–365
89. Hansen EK. After polymerization of visible light-activated resins: surface hardness vs light source. Scan J Dent Res 1983; 91:406–410
90. Watts DC, McNaughton V, Grant AA. The development of surface hardness in visible light-cured posterior composites. J Dent 1986; 14:169–174
91. Johnson WM, Leung RL, Fan PL. A mathematical model for post-irradiation hardening of photo-activated composite resins. Dent Mater 1985; 1:191–194
92. Braem M, Lambrechts P, VanHerle G, Davidson CL. Stiffness increase during the setting of dental composite resins. J Dent Res 1987; 66:1713–1716
93. Odén A, Ruyter IE, Øysaed H. Creep and recovery of composites for use in posterior teeth during static and dynamic compression. Dent Mater 1988; 3:147–150
94. Oster G, Yang N. Photopolymerisation of vinyl monomers. Chem Rev 1968; 68:125–151
95. Odian GG. Principles of polymerization. Wiley, New York, 1981
96. Cook WD. Photopolymerization kinetics of dimethacrylates using the camphorquinone amine initiator system. Polymer 1992; 33:600–609
97. Burns W, Dainton F. Two factors affecting the use of the rotating sector in photochemical experiments. Trans Faraday Soc 1950; 46:411
98. Watts DC. Kinetic mechanisms of visible-light-cured resins and resin composites. In: Proc Setting Mechanisms of Dental Materials. Cameron House, Loch Lomond, Scotland, 1992, pp 1–26
99. Watts DC, Cash AJ. Kinetic measurements of photo-polymerisation contraction in resins and composites. Meas Sci Technol 1991; 2:788–794
100. Watts DC, Cash AJ. Determination of polymerization kinetics in visible-light cured materials: methods development. Dent Mater 1991; 7:281–287
101. Andrzejewska E. Photopolymerization kinetics of multifunctional monomers. 2001; 26: 605–665
102. Davidson CL. Conflicting interests with posterior use of composite materials. In: Vanherle G, Smith DC, eds. Posterior composite resin dental restorative materials. Peter Szulc, Amsterdam, 1985, pp 61–65
103. Davidson CL, de Gee AJ. Relaxation of polymerisation contraction stresses by flow in dental composites. J Dent Res 1984; 63:146–148
104. Suliman AA, Boyer DR, Lakes RS. Polymerisation shrinkage of composite resins: comparison with tooth deformation. J Pros Dent 1994; 71:7–12
105. Dauvillier B, Aarnts M, Feilzer A. Developments in shrinkage control of adhesive restoratives. J Esthet Dent 2000; 12:291–299
106. Feilzer AJ, De Gee AJ, Davidson CL. Curing contraction of composites and glass-ionomer cements. J Pros Dent 1988; 59:297–300
107. Miyazaki M, Hinoura K, Onose H, Moore BK. Effect of filler content of light-cured composites on bond strength to bovine dentine. J Dent Res 1991; 19:301–303
108. Culbertson BM, Wan QC, Tong YH. Preparation and evaluation of visible light-cured multi-methacrylates for dental composites. J Macromol Sci Pure Appl Chem A 1997; 34:2405–2421
109. Davy KW, Kalachandra S, Pandain MS, Braden M. Relationship between composite matrix molecular structure and properties. Biomaterials 1998; 19:2007–2014
110. Feilzer A, de Gee A, Davidson C. Setting stress in composite resin in relation to configuration of the restoration. J Dent Res 1987; 66:1636–1639
111. Feilzer AJ, De Gee AJ, Davidson CL. Quantitative determination of stress reduction by flow in composite resin restorations. Dent Mater 1990; 6:167–171
112. Choi KK, Condon JR, Ferracane JL. The effects of adhesive thickness on polymerisation contraction stress of composite. J Dent Res 2000; 79:812–817

113. Chen H, Manhart J, Kunzelmann K-H, Hickel R. Polymerization contraction stress in light-cured compomer restorative materials. Dent Mater 2003; 19:597–602
114. Armstrong S, Keller J, Boyer D. The influence of water storage and C-factor on the dentin–resin composite microtensile bond strength and debond pathway utilizing a filled and unfilled adhesive resin. Dent Mater 2001; 17:268–276
115. Bouillaguet S, Ciucchi B, Jacoby T, Wataha J, Pashley D. Bonding characteristics to dentin walls of class II cavities, in vitro. Dent Mater 2001; 17:316–321
116. Loguercio A, Reisa A, Ballester R. Polymerization shrinkage: effects of constraint and filling technique in composite restorations. Dent Mater 2004; 20:236–243
117. Prati C, Nucci C, Davidson CL, Montanari G. Early marginal leakage and shear bond strength of adhesive restorative systems. Dent Mater 1990; 6:195–200
118. Retief DH, O'Brien JA, Smith LA, Marchman JL. In vitro investigation and evaluation of dentin bonding agents. Am J Dent 1988; 1:176–183
119. Bandyopadhyay S. A study of the volumetric setting shrinkage of some dental materials. J Biomed Mater Res 1982; 16:135–144
120. Venhoven BAM, de Gee AJ, Davidson CL. Polymerization contraction and conversion of light-curing bisGMA-based methacrylate resins. Biomaterials 1993; 14:871–875
121. de Boer J, Visser R, Melis G. Time-resolved determination of volume shrinkage and refractive index change of volume shrinkage and refractive index change of thin polymer films during photopolymerization. Polymer 1992; 33:1123–1126
122. Ensaff H, O'Docherty D, Jacobsen P. Polymerization shrinkage of dental composite resins. Proc Inst Mech Engrs 2001; 215:367–375
123. Shlesinger MF. Williams-Watts dielectric relaxation: a fractal time stochastic process. J Stat Phys 1984; 36:639–648
124. Williams G, Watts DC. Non-symmetrical dielectric relaxation behaviour arising from a simple empirical decay function. Trans Faraday Soc 1970; 66:80–85
125. Braga R, Ferracane J. Contraction stress related to degree of conversion and reaction kinetics. J Dent Res 2002; 81:114–118
126. Loshaek S, Fox T. Cross-linked polymers. I. Factors influencing the efficiency of cross-linking in copolymers of methyl methacylate and glycol dimethacrylate. J Am Chem Soc 1953; 75:3544–3550
127. Patel MP, Braden M, Davy KWM. Polymerisation shrinkage of methacrylate esters. Biomaterials 1987; 8:53–56
128. Gilbert J, Hasenwinkel J, Wixson R, Lautenschlager E. A theoretical and experimental analysis of polymerization shrinkage of bone cement: a potential major source of porosity. J Biomed Mater Res 2000; 52:210–218
129. Rose E, Lal J, Green R. Effects of peroxide, amine and hydroquinone in varying concentrations on the polymerization rate of polymethyl methacrylate slurries. J Am Dent Assoc 1958; 56:375–381
130. Castille YP. Physical properties of monomers. The polymer handbook, 1st edn. In: Brandrup J, Immergut E, McDowell W, eds. Wiley, New York, 1975, section VIII-16
131. Silikas N, Al-Kheraif A, Watts DC. Influence of P/L ratio and peroxide/amine concentrations on shrinkage-strain kinetics during setting of PMMA/MMA biomaterial formulations. Biomaterials 2005; 26:197–204
132. Asmussen E, Peutzfeldt A. Influence of pulse-delay curing on softening of polymer structures. J Dent Res 2001; 80:1570–1573
133. Watts DC, Marouf AS, El Hejazi A, Al Hindi A, Ibrahim A. Evolution of shrinkage and expansion stresses in dental resin composites. Proc Soc Exper Mech 2001:96–98
134. Watts DC, Marouf AS, Al Hindi AM. Photo-polymerization shrinkage-stress kinetics in resin-composites at standardized compliance: methods development. Dent Mater 2002; 18
135. Thompson VP, Williams EF, Bailey WJ. Dental resins with reduced shrinkage during hardening. J Dent Res 1979; 58:1522–1532

Bonding in Prosthodontics with Cements 7

A. El Zohairy, A.J. Feilzer

Introduction

When a tooth becomes decayed or fractured, an indirect restoration may be indicated to restore its functional and biological integrity. To reach that goal, special requirements have to be set for the properties of the cement used to retain the restoration. From a biological point of view the health of the pulp has to be ensured by the creation of a tight and durable seal of the dentinal tubules, whereas from a mechanical point of view that seal has to resist the forces caused by functional loading of the restoration and the stresses caused by dimensional changes during cement setting and use. Moreover, the optical properties of the restorative system, which includes the cement and the restorative material, should correspond to that of the tooth to create an esthetic restoration of high quality; thus, the key for the success of any restorative dental material depends on its ability to fulfill simultaneously biological, mechanical, and esthetic requirements to guarantee the health of the tooth, periodontal tissues, and the surrounding tissues, as well as patient satisfaction.

In the past the function of the dental cements relied mainly on the mechanical requirements, and the creation of retention by simply filling the gap between the restoration and tooth structure. The retentive quality of these non-adhesive cements depends on the amount of friction generated between the restoration and the preferably prepared parallel walls and the mechanical strength of the cement. If applicable, supplementary retention can also be added by means of grooves, skirts, slots, pins, or dowels. From a biological point of view the preservation of tooth health with those conventional non-adhesive cements is more or less limited to an attempt to minimize the entrance of fluids by filling the space between the restoration and the preparation. As the thickness of remaining dentin after preparation is inversely proportional to the pulpal response, minimal preparation is advised; however, to achieve sufficient mechanical retention the operator has to remove sound tooth structure that subsequently may lead to a harmful pulpal effect and unduly will weaken the remaining tooth structure. Moreover, dentin crazing or root fracture could develop from the use of supplementary retentive means such as pins and radicular posts [1, 2]. The use of cements with adhesive properties may give dentistry a tool to overcome these problems, as bonding the restorative material to the underlying tooth structure makes, in contrast to the use of non-adhesive cements, a less invasive restorative approach. With these cements biomechanical preservation of sound tooth tissue became possible. Not only the extra retentive possibilities but also a durable sealing of the dentin "wound" comes into view with adhesive cements. Biologically, adhesive cements should be not only non-irritant to the pulp–dentin complex and the surrounding soft tissues but also seal the tooth restoration interface to prevent microleakage and the potential subsequent ingress of microorganisms. Microleakage and ingress of microorganisms is considered to be the main etiological factor for pulpal damage; therefore, an effective and durable seal of the tubules should be aimed, as it will enhance the longevity of the pulp vitality. This goal is easier reached with adhesive cements than with conventional, non-adhesive cements. The use of adhesive cements opens also a new area in restorative dentistry in which ceramic and resin composite restorative materials can be combined with contemporary adhesives, which enables the dentist to create restorations with improved optical characteristics. These challenges of the application of adhesive technology have had an enormous influence on prosthetic dentistry. Finally, this leads to the increase of patient demands for esthetic restorations, too.

In this chapter we discuss the advantages and the properties of some contemporary adhesive cements, with particular attention on the resin-based cements and their significance for bonding indirect esthetic restorations.

Luting Cements

Originally the term cement was used in dentistry for the restorative and luting materials that are composed of a powder and a liquid. Later, when other delivery systems became popular, materials with equal compositions became available as paste, too. Nevertheless, the development of dental cements can be characterized by the powders and liquids used to make them. The powder is used as cement reinforcing filler and consists mainly of metal oxides (glass, ceramics, zinc oxide), or pre-polymerized resin (polymethyl-methacrylate). The liquid functions as base that forms during the setting reaction a matrix in which the filler particles are embedded and bonded to (Table 7.1). Generally, two types of chemical reactions are recognized: firstly, a polymerization reaction of the resin matrix, initiated by mixing a catalyst with an initiator or by exposing a photo-initiator with light with a wavelength in the range of approximately 470 or 415 nm; and secondly, an acid–base reaction between the basic glass and the acid liquid. Nevertheless, the acid–base reaction of glass-ionomer cements can be interpreted as a type of polymerization reaction as it forms a polymer matrix of polyacrylic acid; thus, nearly all dental luting cements can be characterized as a composite consisting of a matrix filled with a reinforcing filler. The filler particle size and distribution is of influence on the viscosity of the unset cement as well as the film thickness that can be reached with the cement.

Yet, most contemporary cements are based on glass filler. For glass-ionomer-based cements the glass should be acid soluble to enable ion discharge to react with the acrylic acid. The liquid component of most cement is responsible for adhesive properties. Generally, cements that contain only a resin need an adhesion promoter to create adhesion to a substrate, whereas, for instance, glass-ionomer-based cements can create a true chemical bond to the dental hard tissues.

Another way to classify dental luting cements is by dividing them into conventional and adhesive cements. The conventional cements or the non-adhesive

Table 7.1. Classification of cements based on general composition

Liquid/powder	Glass/ceramic	Zn O	Pre-polymerized resin powder[b]
Phosphoric acid	Silicate cement	Zinc phosphate cement	
Acrylic acid	Glass-ionomer cement	Zinc polycarboxylate cement	
Eugenol		Zinc oxide–eugenol cement	
Resin	Resin-composite cement		
Resin and phosphoric acid	Glass phosphonate cement		
Resin and acrylic acid	Resin-modified glass ionomer		
MMA monomer[a]			Unfilled Resin cement

[a] Methyl-methacrylate monomer.
[b] For example, polymethyl-methacrylate polymer.

cements are cements that do not have the potentiality to bond to tooth structure. The "adhesive" luting cements can be divided into two main groups, that of cements that have the intrinsic property to create chemical bonding to the tooth tissues through ionic exchange, and that of cements that can obtain this bond principally by micromechanical interlocking with the conditioned tooth structure. The first group consists mainly of glass-ionomer cements and resin-modified glass-ionomer cement. The second group consists mainly of resin-based cements, which include unfilled adhesive resin cements and composite resin cements. The composite resin cements generally are composed of polyfunctional dimethacrylate-based monomers, such as Bis-GMA and/or urethane dimethacrylate, and inorganic filler of fine glass or ceramic and silica. In other words, their composition is analogous to that of resin-composite restoratives but with a lower filler loading. Actually, in the latter group the adhesive properties are determined by the type of the combined adhesive system and not primarily by the choice of the cement per se. Concern is often raised regarding the risk of pre-curing the bonding agent prior to the insertion of the luting composite on the fit of the indirect restorations. To solve this problem, several ways are possible, firstly, by taking the impression of the prepared tooth after the application and light curing of a bonding agent, and secondly, by utilizing dual-curing bonding agents that do not necessitate separate light curing before cementation. Finally, this problem can be solved by using resin-composite cements that do not need separate adhesion promoters as they utilize self-etching primers and inherent adhesive promoter monomers in the resin component of the lute itself, e.g., Panavia F cement and Bistite II DC cement.

The unfilled resin cements, on the other hand, performs as both the adhesive system and the luting media; hence, for these cements a diffusion promoter monomer is often added to the liquid of the cement, which enables the infiltration

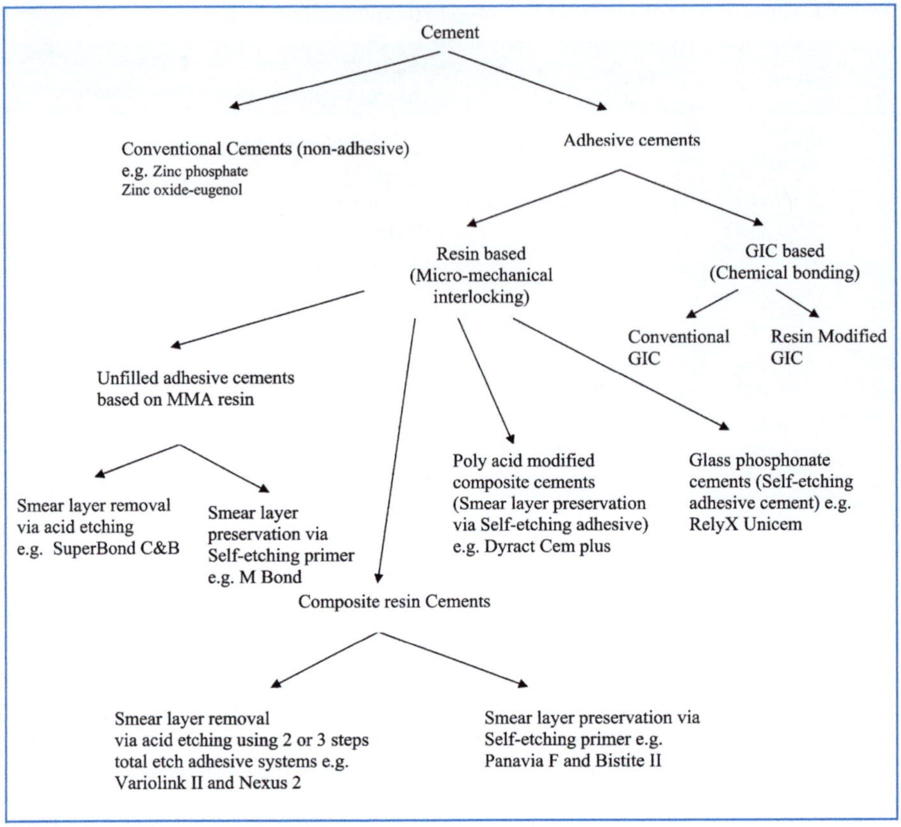

Fig. 7.1. Classification of Luting cements based on adhesion mechanism to tooth structure

of the conditioned dentin. This diffusion promoter is a bifunctional molecule containing hydrophilic and hydrophobic groups. Although the strength of unfilled resin cements is inferior to that of composite resin cements, they have the advantage of being bonded directly to the tooth structure without needing a separate bonding-agent step that might compromise the restoration's fit. In addition, unfilled adhesive resin cements based on MMA monomer are more elastic than those made of polyfunctional, cross-linked polymer chains. The most widespread example of unfilled adhesive resin cement based on MMA monomers is the 4-META/MMA-TBB resin cement (Super-Bond C&B, Sun Medical or C&B Metabond, Parkell). Figure 7.1 gives an overview of the classification of luting cements.

Strength and Solubility

Strength and solubility of the cement is an important parameter for the longevity of the cemented restoration. The conventional zinc ortho-phosphate cements were prone to dissolve in saliva. For that reason a small cement film thickness at the margin is attempted for these cements. Despite the fact that resin-based cements do loose some of their contents when exposed to water, they are hardly soluble; therefore, a very tight fit of restoration cemented with the latter resins is not mandatory. When the cement margins are in the occlusal area, the cement may be prone to occlusal wear. For that reason highly filled cements may be required. As the filler content and size influences the viscosity of the unset cement negatively, special composite cements are developed the viscosity of which can be temporarily lowered by applying ultrasound energy on the restoration to be placed utilizing its thixotropic properties.

Stability and Stiffness

All cements in dentistry do undergo dimensional changes during and after setting. During setting the closer distance between reacted molecules does cause a setting shrinkage, whereas the exposure of the set cement to the oral environment may result in water sorption and swelling. As a reliable bond of the cement to the substrates is attempted, both dimensional changes may lead to stress development at the cement substrate interface. Generally, the setting shrinkage stresses may place the adhesion at risk, whereas the hygroscopic expansion may affect the integrity of all-ceramic restorations. Also, the modulus of elasticity of the cement is of importance for mainly the brittle all-ceramic restorations. Ceramic restorations need a stiff cement, such as resin-composite cement, for providing good support. In contrast, the low modulus of elasticity of the unfilled MMA-based adhesive resin cement offers resiliency and flexibility to the bond with higher resistance to occlusal impact stresses, which is more relevant for splinting loose teeth or cementing adhesive bridges.

Bonding to Tooth Structure

Buonocore in 1955 showed that etching enamel with phosphoric acid leads to loss of superficial enamel with preferential dissolution of the underlying enamel leading to the creation of microporosities [3]. By applying unfilled bonding resins to the etched enamel, the resin can be drawn by capillary attraction into the microporosities to form a resin–enamel interlocked composite layer. This bond is still one of the most reliable; however, the development of self-etching primers and adhesives that require the omitting of the separate etching step may result in insufficient resin–enamel bond due to the weak acidity of some mild self-etching systems. This concern is more relevant when there is a large surface enamel–adhesive interface area such as facial laminate veneers or adhesive bonded-bridge restorations. To tackle this drawback, application of the self-etching primer during a sufficiently long time of at least 15 s and actively applying it through rubbing the enamel surface with repeated applications of fresh material is suggested [4]. Alternatively, a separate step of acid-etching procedure can be accomplished prior to the application of the self-etching primer.

In contrast to bonding to enamel, bonding to dentin is more technically sensitive and is affected by several variables. After preparation of dentin, nearly always

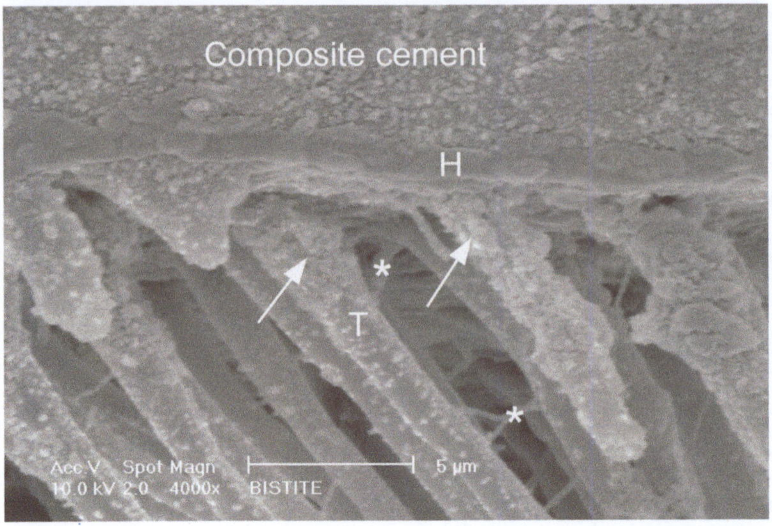

Fig. 7.2. Scanning electron microscopy photomicrograph of resin–dentin interface produced by Bistite-II cement which utilizes self-etching primer. The luting composite is attached to the dentin surface by an acid-resistant hybrid layer (*H*) of 0.6–1 µm. The hybrid layer is extended into the tubule wall forming tubule-wall hybridization (*arrow*) at the top of the resin tags (*T*). Lateral branches (*asterisk*) are formed from the main resin tags representing the high infiltration potentiality of that cement.

a smear layer, consisting of inorganic material and embedded in organic matrix, develops. The layer tenaciously adheres to the prepared dentin surface. For that reason the smear layer and the underlying dentin has to be conditioned to enable resin to penetrate or remove the smear layer and to bond to the underlying dentin. Resin-based adhesive systems utilize different methods to condition dentin. The first method attempts to remove the smear layer completely via acid etching and rinsing. The second approach aims at preservation of the smear layer; however, in both approaches the adhesion is based on micromechanical interlocking by creating a so-called hybrid layer. Among the contemporary adhesive systems are cements that employ self-etching primers that are based on the latter approach (Fig. 7.2). The use of these adhesive systems is an outcome of efforts made to simplify the bonding procedure and to improve the bonding quality by reducing the number of required steps in the bonding procedure. When applied to smear layers, these resin systems demineralize the smear layer and incorporate it into the applied resin, which slightly penetrates into the underlying dentin, thereby creating a hybrid layer in which the undissolved collagen fibers of the dentin are incorporated and which contain the remnants of the original smear layer [5]; thus, the separate steps of using an acid and primer are combined in one procedure. Moreover, a number of contemporary adhesive resin-based cements that utilize self-etching primers do not make use of the separate resin-bonding-agent phase that might affect the fitting of the indirect restorations. More recently, self-etching adhesive resin-based cement was developed (RelyX Unicem, 3 M ESPE). The organic matrix of this cement consists of multifunctional phosphoric acid-modified (meth)-acrylates. This adhesive cement does not employ pretreatment of the tooth surfaces as it depends on the inherent acidity of the resin matrix to condition the tooth surface. The Unicem cement can be categorized as glass phosphonate cement as it is related to silicate cements due to the incorporation of basic inorganic filler within the matrix which participates in the cement reactions together with the acidic groups of the monomer.

Nevertheless, resin cements that utilize self-etching approach generally suffer from the weak acidity of their acidic resin in comparison with phosphoric acid; therefore, it is widely believed that the bonding performance of these systems could be affected by the quantity and quality of the smear layer [6]. Clinicians routinely use diamond burs for extracoronal preparations followed by impression taking and provisional restoration using temporary cements. It was found that bond strength to dentin prepared with diamond burs and conditioned with self-etching primers was lower than that prepared with fine-fissure steel burs and conditioned with the same system. Alternatively, the reduction in bond strength was not observed when the smear layer created by different burs was removed with adhesives that utilize phosphoric acid conditioning [7]. For these reasons, it might be useful to finish the preparation steel burs.

Bonding to Ceramic

Bonding of adhesive resin cement to ceramic can be achieved through micromechanical and/or chemical bonding mechanisms. There are several methods to condition ceramic surfaces to enhance bonding to resin-luting cements, although the effects of different surface treatments on bonding are strongly dependent on the type and the microstructure of the ceramic surface to which to bond [8–10].

Surface Preparation

Mechanical bonding to ceramic surfaces can be enhanced by preparing the surface by grinding, abrasion with a diamond rotary instrument, airborne-particle abrasion with aluminum oxide, and etching using different types of acids. Hydrofluoric acid (HF) is commonly used to etch porcelain for indirect restorations [11, 12]. As alternatives, to avoid the hazardous HF, acidulated phosphate fluoride [8] or phosphoric acid (H_3PO_4) were also used to condition the ceramic surfaces; however, their effectiveness on the enhancement of the bond strength is still doubtful [13]. Phosphoric acid is used in industry to etch glass at high temperature. At room temperature the action of H_3PO_4 is limited to clean the ceramic surface without producing an apparent etching pattern (Fig. 7.3), and therefore this treatment does not contribute to the resin ceramic bond strength [14].

The capability of HF to alter the ceramic surface depends on the ceramic microstructure and composition. Ceramic that contains a glass phase (leucite, silica-based feldspath, or glass ceramics) can be etched with HF, whereas all-ceramic restorations made of aluminous cores cannot be etched sufficiently. The HF creates a surface pattern for micromechanical attachment by preferential dissolution

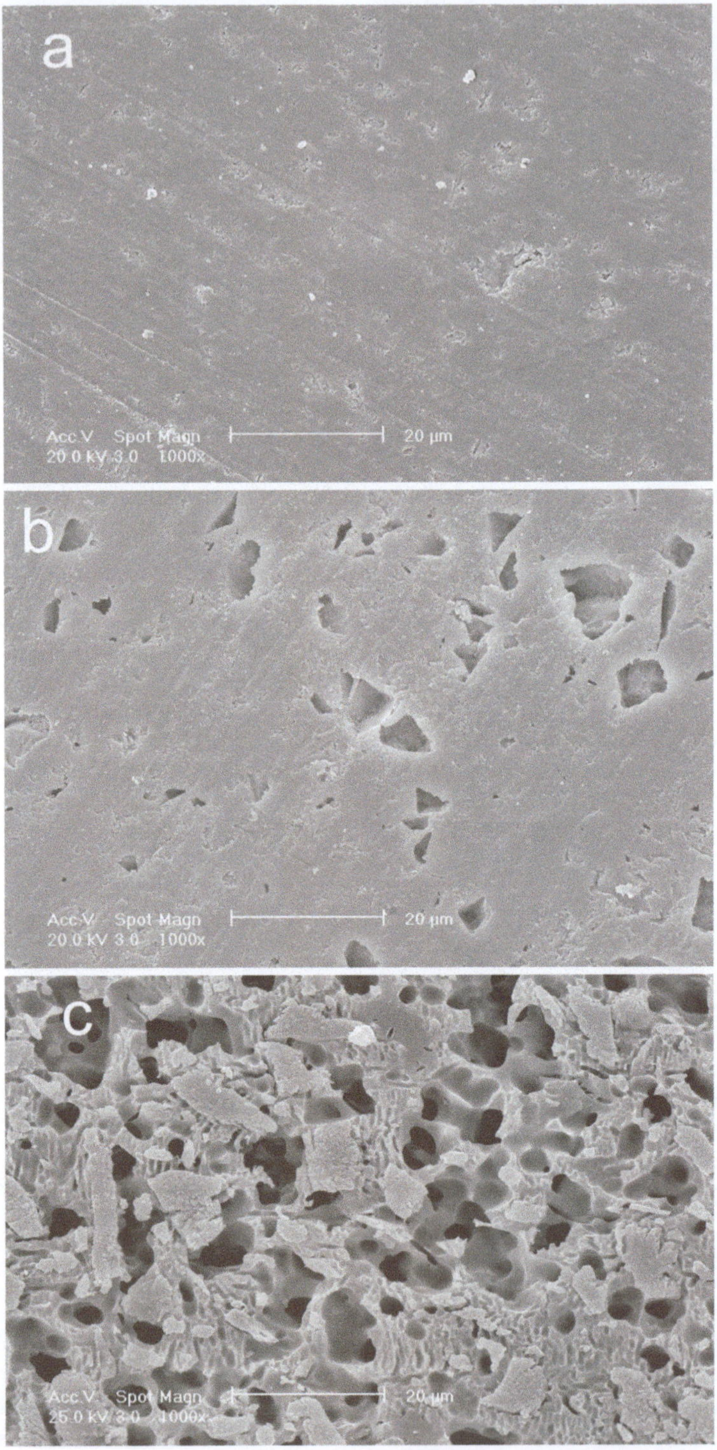
a
Acc.V Spot Magn
20.0 kV 3.0 1000x
20 µm
b
Acc.V Spot Magn
20.0 kV 3.0 1000x
20 µm
c
Acc.V Spot Magn
25.0 kV 3.0 1000x
20 µm

Fig. 7.3 a–c. Scanning electron micrographs of the Vita blocs Mark-II ceramic surfaces. **a** Specimen after 600-grit SiC wet grinding. **b** Specimen treated with 37% H_3PO_4. Note that there are no apparent etching patterns; the surface shows only exposed surface porosities and defects caused by the cleaning action of the acid. **c** Specimen treated with 8% HF. The etching pattern with numerous undercuts for micromechanical retention is clearly seen

of the glass phase from the ceramic matrix which increases the surface area and enhances the micromechanical retention of the resin cement [15]. The micro-undercuts formed on the ceramic surface by HF etching allow the penetration of both the resin and filler components of the luting composite cement to form particle-reinforced resin tags that contribute to strong resin–ceramic bond [16]. Due to this ability of the filler to penetrate the micro-undercuts without being filtered, the resin ceramic bond strength can substantially increase by treating the etched ceramic with filled bonding agent [17]. On the other hand, over-etching with high HF concentrations or extended etching times may lead to a reduced bond strength [18], or HF can be so aggressive to the surface of some ceramic materials that it declines its mechanical properties, which would in turn affect the resin–ceramic bond strength [9, 19]. Consequently, one should take into account the type of ceramic being used before HF etching.

Alumina blasting is used to remove refractory investment material during the laboratory procedures of the fired ceramic restorations when the hot-press technology is used. For these cases the ceramic surface is always gently roughened. It was found that the bond strength of porcelain laminate veneer was greater when etched than when lightly sandblasted [12]. Conversely, excessive sandblasting to improve the bond can induce chipping and adversely affect the fit of all-ceramic restorations without significantly improving bond strength [20, 21].

Chemical Bonding

For effective and durable resin ceramic bond, not only micromechanical bonding, but also a chemical bonding, should be attempted. The most common and effective way to achieve a chemical resin–ceramic bond is through using silane coupling agents. Silane coupling agents are bifunctional molecules that improve the wettability of the ceramic surface and form a covalent bond with both the ceramic and the resin cement [22]. Silane agents commonly consist of γ-methacryloxypropyl trimethoxysilane (γ-MPTS). The reaction between methoxy silane groups of γ-MPTS and OH groups of the porcelain surface that formed siloxane bonds can be initiated and accelerated by using acid catalysis [23]. Presently, contemporary ceramic primers utilize separate acidic catalyst liquids, such as monomer of 10-methacryloyloxydecyl dihydrogen phosphate (MDP), or carboxylic compound. When the acidic catalyst is mixed with the silane coupler component, the methoxyl groups hydrolyze to initiate stable siloxane bond (Si–O–Si) with the porcelain surface (Fig. 7.4) [24].

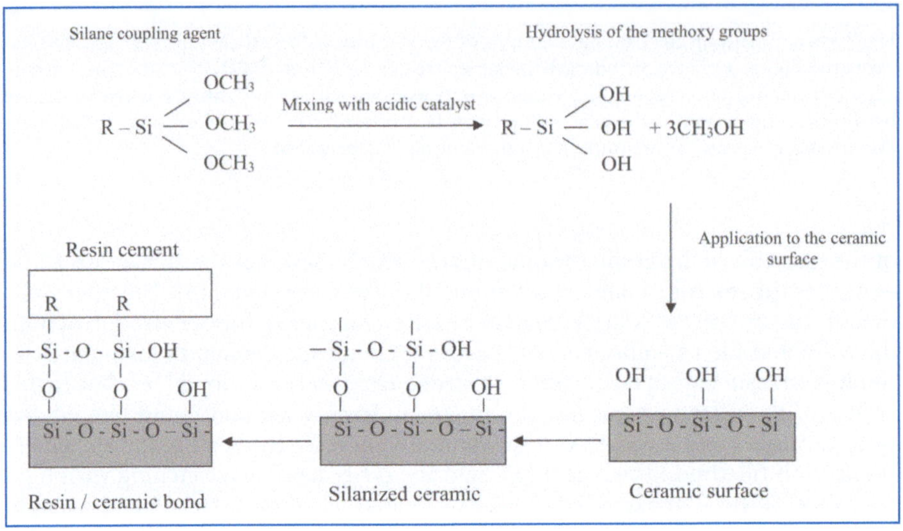

Fig. 7.4. Silane treatment procedure

Accordingly, ceramic primers can be classified as follows [25]:
1. Unhydrolyzed single-liquid silane primer
2. Prehydrolyzed silane primer that is also single liquid
3. Two- or three-liquid primer with separate silane coupler and acid activator

The single-liquid prehydrolyzed silane primer has shown a better bonding performance than the unhydrolyzed form; however, the stability of the prehydrolyzed silane primer appears to be insufficient and its shelf life is limited compared with the multicomponent liquid primers [25].

Improvement in ceramic resin bond strength can also be accomplished through heat treatment of the silanized porcelain. It is believed that during heating (100 °C for 60 s) water and other contaminates, such as alcohol or acetic acid, are eliminated from the silane-treated surface, which drives the silane/silica surface condensation reaction towards completion and promotes silane silica bond formation [21].

The try-in procedure is an important step for all-ceramic restoration to optimize fitting and color match. Etching and silane treatment are best accomplished after the try-in procedure to prevent contamination of the conditioned ceramic surface. Nevertheless, for the convenience of dental practitioners, to save time at the chair side, many commercial dental laboratories etch and silanize the fitting surface of the ceramic restoration. When this pretreated surface is contaminated during the try-in procedure, with saliva or blood, the surface has to be cleaned and silanized again before the application of the adhesive cement. Cleaning can be carried out with phosphoric acid or acetone, after which time the silane treatment has to be repeated [26].

Due to the high concentration of various solvents within the silane-coupling agents, an improperly sealed container will permit evaporation of the solvent, which increases the concentration of coupling agent, which in turn can act as a separation medium and adversely affects the resin–ceramic bond strength [27].

Although many laboratory studies have shown that only silane treatment without additional micromechanical bonding could provide sufficient resin–ceramic bond strength [23, 28], the technical sensitivity of silane treatment and the complicated multi-step cementing procedure favor employing the twofold bonding mechanism to insure strong and durable bond.

Nevertheless, HF etching followed by silanization, which enhances the resin bond to conventional silica-based ceramics, does not improve the resin bond strength to alumina- or zirconia-based ceramics. This is probably due to the inherent microstructure of the latter ceramics, which are more resistant to the HF acid. Moreover, as a consequence of the small percentage of silica at the surface of alumina-based ceramics and its nonexistence in the zirconia ceramics, it is less likely that silane treatment can initiate effective chemical bonding. Tribochemical application of a silica layer by means of sandblasting (Rocatec system, 3 M ESPE, Seefeld, Germany) followed by silane application was found to provide long-term durable bond of BIS-GMA composite resin cement to alumina-based ceramic [29]. In addition, the ability of the phosphate ester group contained in some adhesive resin-based cement (e.g., Panavia cements) to bond directly to metal oxides can also offer an alternative bonding mechanism to sandblasted alumina-based or zirconia ceramics.

Bonding to Pre-Processed Composite Restorations

The first composite inlays were made from a microfilled material, which was heat-and-pressed cured [30], followed by an inlay system based on a light-cured hybrid composite (DI system, Coltène, Switzerland), which was launched in 1987. The secondary heat cure which is included during fabrication of the pre-processed composite restoration increases the rate of monomer conversion and enhances cross-linking which results in improved physical and mechanical properties [31, 32]; however, bonding of resin cements to pre-processed composite restorations may be challenged by the reduced number of reactive sites due to the high degree of double-bond conversion. For this reason the bonded surface of the pre-processed composite should be mechanical and chemically modified to improve bonding of the resin cement. Similarly to all-ceramic restorations, the capability of HF to alter the pre-processed composite surface is generally influenced by the nature of the reinforcing filler. The HF has been shown to improve bond strength to microfilled composite inlays, as it has a roughening effect by preferentially attacking the SiO_2 glass filler [33]. An additional silane treatment of the surface would further enhance the bond strength, as mainly the filler particles at the surface are potential sites for silanization and the well-cured resin matrix does not provide much remaining double C=C bonds to bond with. In contrast, HF has an aggressive etching effect over glass-filled hybrid composites which can degrade partially the resin matrix and cause total dissolution of exposed glass filler particles with subsequent deterioration in resin bond strength [34, 35]. It seems that the most effective method to enhance bonding to pre-processed composite is one which employs roughening of the bonded surface followed by the application of a coating of an intermediate bonding agent [17, 36–38].

Biological Considerations

At the present time biological seal of cut tooth tissues can be achieved either through auto-adhesion mechanisms by ionic bond formation using glass-ionomer-based cement or through micromechanical interlocking of adhesive resin-based cements with the tooth tissues by forming an impermeable resin-infiltrated hybrid layer [39]. Adhesively retained restorations yield profit in terms of the conservation of sound tooth structure especially with teeth of compromised retention due to short, over-convergent, or insufficient remaining tooth to retain a restoration. Additionally, by relying on the bonding potentiality of the adhesive cements, it is more feasible to end the preparation line above the gingival margin, which ensures minimal periodontal response.

It is important for the cement–tooth interface to maintain strong adhesion, not only for resistance to early marginal alteration, due to the dimensional changes of the material during setting, but also for a durable seal to resist bacterial acidic attack and the oral detrimental factors. However, an absolute leak-proof and durable, strong resin dentin bond could thus far not be reached [40–44]; therefore, a luting cement which is able to release fluoride may play a role in caries inhibition, which is of value for the leaking parts of the cement–tooth interface. For this to occur a strong initial fluoride release "burst effect," and a less strong, stable, and constant release are required from the material in order to reduce caries activity [45]. It has been reported that glass-ionomer cement and resin-modified glass ionomer showed an initial higher fluoride burst effect and higher fluoride uptake in comparison with polyacid-modified and fluoride-containing composite [46–49]; however, the low mechanical strength and the moisture sensitivity of the conventional glass-ionomer cement and the high water sorption tendency of the resin-modified glass-ionomer cements limits their ability to be used as adhesive cements particularly for retaining all-ceramic restorations.

Mechanical Considerations

Metal and porcelain-fused-to-metal restorations have for a long time been successfully luted with non-adhesive cements. The main additional merit of using adhesive cementation for metal ceramic restorations is to give extra retention for preparations with compromised retention, although using resin-adhesive cements with relatively high film thickness could disturb the accurate placement of the restoration. In contrast, the brittle nature of all-ceramic restoration requires the use of strong stable substructure to support the restoration against the destructive tensile stresses. This goal can be reached either by a strong adhesion of the ceramic to the metal support or adhesive bonding the ceramic with the underlying tooth structure. Various investigations have shown that all-ceramic restorations cemented with adhesive resin-based cements have higher fracture resistance when compared with non-adhesive cemented restorations [50, 51]. It is believed that the bonding capability of the adhesive resin cement is able to repair the surface flaws located at the fitting surface of the all-ceramic restoration; hence, it might reduce the potential for crack propagation. Besides, the higher fracture toughness and improved mechanical properties of resin-based cement, in comparison with conventional cements, enables it to create better support and load transfer through the brittle ceramic restoration to the underlying tooth structure [52].

On the other hand, conventional glass-ionomer cement suffers from low mechanical properties and low bonding capability to ceramic material that can lead to failure and marginal breakdown of the ceramic inlays under occlusal loading [53]. The clinical efficacy of the resin-based luting cement over a glass ionomer for cementing ceramic restoration has also been reported [54–56]. Resin-modified glass-ionomer cements were developed to overcome these specific disadvantages of conventional glass-ionomer cements, and increased values of fracture toughness have been reported for restorative-grade cements; however, a major concern about using resin-modified glass-ionomer cement for bonding all-ceramic restorations is its hygroscopic expansion. Although all glass-ionomer cements do shrink during setting, after being set, they show expansion due to water uptake from the surrounding environment. This expansion is more pronounce and excessive with resin modified glass-ionomer cements due to the high water sorption tendency of the hydrophilic resin component of the cement; therefore, the cemented all-ceramic restoration may come under an expansion stress, which increases the risk for crack propagation [57] and failure. For the purpose of maintaining a strong cement–tooth and cement–ceramic bond, the dimensional stability of the adhesive cement during and after setting is crucial. The setting of resin-based cements takes place after initiation of the polymerization reaction of the matrix phase. The conversion of the monomer molecules into a polymer network is accompanied with a closer packing of the molecules, which leads to a reduction of volume [58] usually denoted as curing contraction or polymerization shrinkage. When the contraction of the adhesive materials is hindered, stresses are induced which can be detrimental for the bonded interfaces or even the cohesive strength of the cement [59]. In cases with an unfavorable configuration (C-factor), where the ratio of bonded surface to free surface of the shrinkage material is higher than five, all shrinkage will be directed uniaxially, leading to a contraction that is almost three times higher than the expected linear shrinkage [10]. Cement films exhibit unfavorable C-factors because the shrinkage of the cement is totally hindered by both the restoration and the tooth interfaces; thus, the initial bond of the shrinkage cement to tooth/restoration interfaces should exceed the contraction stresses. However, some stress relief may originate from the surrounding structures, as for the thin cement film only a small amount of compensation by shrinkage strain of the restoration and/or the cavity walls may be enough to drop down the developing shrinkage stresses to a level lower than the adhesive strength of the cement at that very moment.

Curing Strategies

Resin-based luting cements can be categorized on the basis of their polymerization method into auto-cure cements, light-cure cements, and dual-cure cements. For facial veneers, light-cured resin cement can be used due to the superior accessibility of that particular restoration. When access of the curing light is limited for large ceramic or resin-composite indirect restorations, dual-cure resin-based cements are recommended to compensate for light attenuation affected by the restoration thickness and shade [60]; however, self-curing alone is insufficient for dual-cured cements to achieve maximum hardening [61, 62]. In the absence of light, polymerizations start by chemical initiation only, which results in poor mechanical properties of the cement and consequently poor bonding potentiality to the restoration; therefore, it is recommended to direct the light-curing tip at the restoration from several directions to insure higher initiation effect to the dual-cure cement by light.

Esthetic Considerations

As the adhesive technology made it possible to create tooth-colored restorations, not only the esthetic requirements of the restorative materials became an issue but also that of the luting cements. In two ways the esthetic properties of the luting cement can be of importance, firstly, its color properties, concerning color translucency and opaqueness, and secondly, the color stability.

Color

Mainly for veneers the color of the cement may influence the final shade of the restoration; however, one has to recognize that a luting cement can never change a wrongly chosen color of an esthetic restoration into a matching color. Only a slight shade change can be reached with luting cements. Mainly the opaqueness of the cement is of importance for cases in which the dentist wants to hide discolored dentin. Also, for these cases the normal thin cement layer will not be able to hide totally such a discoloration.

It is important for two reasons to know the type of photo-initiator in resin-based restoratives used to lute esthetic restorations, as the yellow color of camphorquinone changes with the curing of the cement into white. Uncured resin-based cements may therefore be more yellow than cured ones. Some cement does contain *bis*-acylphosphine oxide (BAPO) as photo-initiator, which does not show this effect; however, BAPO does not cure at light with a wave length of 470 nm but of 415 nm. Most LED-based curing lights do not cover this wavelength range and cannot be used to cure the BAPO-containing cements.

Color Stability

Cements may discolor during lifetime due to the absorption of dyes from food. Two properties are of importance for the sensitivity of cured cements to this discoloration. The degree of cure has an important influence on the color stability: an improper cure makes resin-based cements prone to discoloration. Also, the hydrophilicity of the resin component of the cement is of influence. The more hydrophilic the resin is, the less color stable the cement. This was the main drawback of the earliest resin-modified glass-ionomer cements that contained HEMA, which is a very hydrophilic acrylate. Generally, the resin-based composite cements are less prone to discoloration, if properly cured, than resin-modified glass-ionomer cements.

Value of the Bond Strength Test

Despite the fact that there are many properties on which the dentist can base a choice of adhesive cement, the manufacturers approach the dentist mainly with impressive data with regard to bonding quality. These data are mostly based on bond strength determination of the cements to tooth tissues.

During the past decade many new bonding systems have been introduced for which good clinical performance is claimed. Such claims have to be proven in laboratory studies as well as clinically; however, it is difficult to predict the clinical success of adhesive systems from only laboratory experiments. Moreover, the rapid shift of the manufacturer from one system to a newly developed one does not provide sufficient time for long-term clinical evaluation.

Many investigators have questioned the reliability of the conventional shear and tensile bond strength tests. There are numerous reports on bond strength evaluation in which tests are applied, not only with different designs, but also showing varying incompatible results between studies using the same design. Furthermore, it has been shown that the type of bond strength test and size of the specimen have a relatively large influence on the test results [63, 64].

A crucial factor in evaluating the usefulness of a specific bond strength test is a thorough awareness of the stress patterns, which are involved in bond failure. For all tests the average bond strength is calculated by dividing the load at fracture by the area of the bonded surface, which in fact is based on the assumption of equal stress distribution at the adhesive interface; however, finite element analysis studies demonstrated that the manner in which loads are generally applied in common shear or tensile bond strength tests results in non-uniform stress patterns [65]. Conventional bond strength tests also suffer from frequent cohesive failures within the bonded substrate, which reflect the discrepancy between the actual cohesive strength of that substrate and the apparent low stress measured [66–68].

As a solution to overcome these problems, the microtensile bond strength test (μTBS test) was introduced [69]. With the μTBS test a reduced incidence of dentin cohesive failures and higher bond strength values were reported in comparison with the more conventional tests. These differences were explained by the reduction of the number and size of flaws, as an outcome of the diminution in specimen size [70]; however, it is unclear why such a wide variance of values are reported by different investigators when employing the μTBS test. In addition, the high bond strength values obtained by using the μTBS should not be interpreted as an outcome of improved bonding capability of a particular system rather than the consequence of an altered test setup. The larger bonding area used with the conventional tensile and shear bond strength tests results in less uniform stress distribution of the applied load in comparison with the smaller bonding areas employed with the μTBS, and hence higher bond strength values generally obtained by the latter test.

Thus far, a clear relationship between the bond strength of an adhesive system and its sealing capacity has still not been established, which brings the validity of using only the bond strength data to predict the adhesion efficiency of the system further into question. It is much more likely that bond strength tests should be used as screening tests to compare one system with another using the same test configuration or to determine the effect of changing some variables within a system [71], even though preferences of one adhesive system over the other on the basis of numerical comparison or using unreliable statistical approach could give misleading conclusions; therefore, it is necessary to utilize reliable and standard laboratory tests combined with short-term controlled clinical studies to predict the efficiency of a particular adhesive system.

Finally, the decision making by the clinician to shift to a new adhesive system should be based principally on his own clinical experience with his current adhesive system and whether or not it is mandatory to change.

References

1. Pontius O, Hutter JW. Survival rate and fracture strength of incisors restored with different post and core systems and endodontically treated incisors without coronoradicular reinforcement. J Endod 2002; 28:710–715
2. Webb EL, Straka WF, Phillips CL. Tooth crazing associated with threaded pins:a three-dimensional model. J Prosthet Dent 1989; 61:624–628
3. Buonocore MG. A simple method of increasing the adhesion of acrylic filling materials to enamel surfaces. J Dent Res 1955; 34:849–853
4. Van Meerbeek B, Vargas M, Inoue S, Yoshida Y, Peumans M, Lambrechts P, Vanherle G. Adhesives and cements to promote preservation dentistry. Oper Dent 2001:119–144
5. Watanabe I, Nakabayashi N, Pashley DH. Bonding to ground dentin by a phenyl-P self-etching primer. J Dent Res 1994; 73:1212–1220
6. Ogata M, Harada N, Yamaguchi S, Nakajima M, Pereira PN, Tagami J. Effects of different burs on dentin bond strengths of self-etching primer bonding systems. Oper Dent 2001; 26:375–382
7. Ogata M, Harada N, Yamaguchi S, Nakajima M, Tagami J. Effect of self-etching primer vs phosphoric acid etchant on bonding to bur-prepared dentin. Oper Dent 2002; 27:447–454
8. Lacy AM, LaLuz J, Watanabe LG, Dellinges M. Effect of porcelain surface treatment on the bond to composite. J Prosthet Dent 1988; 60:288–291
9. Della Bona A, Anusavice KJ, Shen C. Microtensile strength of composite bonded to hot-pressed ceramics. J Adhes Dent 2000; 2:305–313
10. Feilzer AJ, De Gee AJ, Davidson CL. Increased wall-to-wall curing contraction in thin bonded resin layers (see comments). J Dent Res 1989; 68:48–50
11. Horn HR. Porcelain laminate veneers bonded to etched enamel. Dent Clin North Am 1983; 27:671–684

12. Calamia JR. Etched porcelain veneers: the current state of the art. Quintessence Int 1985; 16:5–12
13. Kato H, Matsumura H, Atsuta M. Effect of etching and sandblasting on bond strength to sintered porcelain of unfilled resin. J Oral Rehabil 2000; 27:103–110
14. El Zohairy A, De Gee AJ, Feilzer A, Davidson CL. Long-term micro-tensile bond strength of resin cements bonded to CAD/CAM ceramic blocks. J Dent Res 2002; 81:380
15. al Edris A, al Jabr A, Cooley RL, Barghi N. SEM evaluation of etch patterns by three etchants on three porcelains. J Prosthet Dent 1990; 64:734–739
16. Peumans M, Van Meerbeek B, Yoshida Y, Lambrechts P, Vanherle G. Porcelain veneers bonded to tooth structure: an ultra-morphological FE-SEM examination of the adhesive interface. Dent Mater 1999; 15:105–119
17. El Zohairy AA, De Gee AJ, Mohsen MM, Feilzer AJ. Microtensile bond strength testing of luting cements to prefabricated CAD/CAM ceramic and composite blocks. Dent Mater 2005; 21:83–93
18. Chen JH, Matsumura H, Atsuta M. Effect of etchant, etching period, and silane priming on bond strength to porcelain of composite resin. Oper Dent 1998; 23:250–257
19. Shimada Y, Yamaguchi S, Tagami J. Micro-shear bond strength of dual-cured resin cement to glass ceramics. Dent Mater 2002; 18:380–388
20. Heymann HO, Bayne SC, Sturdevant JR, Wilder AD Jr, Roberson TM. The clinical performance of CAD-CAM-generated ceramic inlays: a 4-year study. J Am Dent Assoc 1996; 127:1171–1181
21. Roulet JF, Soderholm KJ, Longmate J. Effects of treatment and storage conditions on ceramic/composite bond strength. J Dent Res 1995; 74:381–387
22. Paffenbarger GC, Sweeney WT, Bowen RL. Bonding porcelain teeth to acrylic resin denture bases. J Am Dent Assoc 1967; 74:1018–1023
23. Aida M, Hayakawa T, Mizukawa K. Adhesion of composite to porcelain with various surface conditions. J Prosthet Dent 1995; 73:464–470
24. Sato K, Matsumura H, Atsuta M. Effect of three-liquid bonding agents on bond strength to a machine-milled ceramic material. J Oral Rehabil 1999; 26:570–574
25. Matsumura H, Kato H, Atsuta M. Shear bond strength to feldspathic porcelain of two luting cements in combination with three surface treatments. J Prosthet Dent 1997; 78:511–517
26. Della Bona A, Northeast SE. Shear bond strength of resin bonded ceramic after different try-in procedures. J Dent 1994; 22:103–107
27. Barghi N. To silanate or not to silanate: making a clinical decision. Compend Contin Educ Dent 2000; 21:659–662, 664; quiz 666
28. Hooshmand T, van Noort R, Keshvad A. Bond durability of the resin-bonded and silane treated ceramic surface. Dent Mater 2002; 18:179–188
29. Kern M, Strub JR. Bonding to alumina ceramic in restorative dentistry: clinical results over up to 5 years. J Dent 1998; 26:245–249
30. James DF, Yarovesky U. An esthetic inlay technique for posterior teeth. Quintessence Int 1983; 14:725–731
31. Wendt SL Jr. The effect of heat used as secondary cure upon the physical properties of three composite resins. II. Wear, hardness, and color stability. Quintessence Int 1987; 18:351–356
32. Wendt SL Jr. The effect of heat used as a secondary cure upon the physical properties of three composite resins. I. Diametral tensile strength, compressive strength, and marginal dimensional stability. Quintessence Int 1987; 18:265–271
33. DeSchepper EJ, Tate WH, Powers JM. Bond strength of resin cements to microfilled composites. Am J Dent 1993; 6:235–238
34. Swift EJ Jr, Brodeur C, Cvitko E, Pires JA. Treatment of composite surfaces for indirect bonding. Dent Mater 1992; 8:193–196
35. Tate WH, DeSchepper EJ, Powers JM. Bond strength of resin cements to a hybrid composite. Am J Dent 1993; 6:195–198
36. Frankenberger R, Strobel WO, Baresel J, Trapper T, Kramer N, Petschelt A. Effect of surface treatment on fatigue behaviour between Tetric Ceram inlays and Variolink luting composite. Clin Oral Investig 2001; 5:260–265

37. Turner CW, Meiers JC. Repair of an aged, contaminated indirect composite resin with a direct, visible-light-cured composite resin. Oper Dent 1993; 18:187–194
38. Latta MA, Barkmeier WW. Bond strength of a resin cement to a cured composite inlay material. J Prosthet Dent 1994; 72:189–193
39. Nakabayashi N, Kojima K, Masuhara E. The promotion of adhesion by the infiltration of monomers into tooth substrates. J Biomed Mater Res 1982; 16:265–273
40. Shono Y, Terashita M, Shimada J, Kozono Y, Carvalho RM, Russell CM, Pashley DH. Durability of resin-dentin bonds. J Adhes Dent 1999; 1:211–218
41. Armstrong SR, Keller JC, Boyer DB. The influence of water storage and C-factor on the dentin–resin composite microtensile bond strength and debond pathway utilizing a filled and unfilled adhesive resin. Dent Mater 2001; 17:268–276
42. Okuda M, Pereira PN, Nakajima M, Tagami J. Relationship between nanoleakage and long-term durability of dentin bonds. Oper Dent 2001; 26:482–490
43. Okuda M, Pereira PN, Nakajima M, Tagami J, Pashley DH. Long-term durability of resin dentin interface: nanoleakage vs microtensile bond strength. Oper Dent 2002; 27:289–296
44. Takahashi A, Inoue S, Kawamoto C, Ominato R, Tanaka T, Sato Y, Pereira PN, Sano H. In vivo long-term durability of the bond to dentin using two adhesive systems. J Adhes Dent 2002; 4:151–159
45. Forsten L. Fluoride release and uptake by glass-ionomers and related materials and its clinical effect. Biomaterials 1998; 19:503–508
46. Forsten L. Resin-modified glass ionomer cements: fluoride release and uptake. Acta Odontol Scand 1995; 53:222–225
47. Forsten L. Fluoride release and uptake by glass ionomers. Scand J Dent Res 1991; 99:241–245
48. Attar N, Onen A. Fluoride release and uptake characteristics of aesthetic restorative materials. J Oral Rehabil 2002; 29:791–798
49. Swift EJ Jr. Fluoride release from two composite resins. Quintessence Int 1989; 20:895–897
50. Burke FJ, Watts DC. Fracture resistance of teeth restored with dentin-bonded crowns. Quintessence Int 1994; 25:335–340
51. Dietschi D, Maeder M, Meyer JM, Holz J. In vitro resistance to fracture of porcelain inlays bonded to tooth. Quintessence Int 1990; 21:823–831
52. Mitchell CA, Douglas WH, Cheng YS. Fracture toughness of conventional, resin-modified glass-ionomer and composite luting cements. Dent Mater 1999; 15:7–13
53. Abdalla AI, Davidson CL. Marginal integrity after fatigue loading of ceramic inlay restorations luted with three different cements. Am J Dent 2000; 13:77–80
54. Aberg CH, van Dijken JW, Olofsson AL. Three-year comparison of fired ceramic inlays cemented with composite resin or glass ionomer cement. Acta Odontol Scand 1994; 52:140–149
55. van Dijken JW, Horstedt P. Marginal breakdown of fired ceramic inlays cemented with glass polyalkenoate (ionomer) cement or resin composite. J Dent 1994; 22:265–272
56. van Dijken JW, Hoglund-Aberg C, Olofsson AL. Fired ceramic inlays: a 6-year follow up. J Dent 1998; 26:219–225
57. Sindel J, Frankenberger R, Kramer N, Petschelt A. Crack formation of all-ceramic crowns dependent on different core build-up and luting materials. J Dent 1999; 27:175–181
58. Venhoven BA, de Gee AJ, Davidson CL. Polymerization contraction and conversion of light-curing BisGMA-based methacrylate resins. Biomaterials 1993; 14:871–875
59. Davidson CL, de Gee AJ. Relaxation of polymerization contraction stresses by flow in dental composites. J Dent Res 1984; 63:146–148
60. Hofmann N, Papsthart G, Hugo B, Klaiber B. Comparison of photo-activation versus chemical or dual-curing of resin-based luting cements regarding flexural strength, modulus and surface hardness. J Oral Rehabil 2001; 28:1022–1028
61. Linden JJ, Swift EJ Jr, Boyer DB, Davis BK. Photo-activation of resin cements through porcelain veneers. J Dent Res 1991; 70:154–157
62. Foxton RM, Pereira PN, Nakajima M, Tagami J, Miura H. Durability of the dual-cure resin cement/ceramic bond with different curing strategies. J Adhes Dent 2002; 4:49–59
63. Phrukkanon S, Burrow MF, Tyas MJ. Effect of cross-sectional surface area on bond strengths between resin and dentin. Dent Mater 1998; 14:120–128

64. Cardoso PE, Braga RR, Carrilho MR. Evaluation of micro-tensile, shear and tensile tests determining the bond strength of three adhesive systems. Dent Mater 1998; 14:394–398
65. Van Noort R, Noroozi S, Howard IC, Cardew G. A critique of bond strength measurements. J Dent 1989; 17:61–67
66. Øilo G, Austrheim EK. In vitro quality testing of dentin adhesives. Acta Odontol Scand 1993; 51:263–269
67. Holtan JR, Nystrom GP, Olin PS, Phelps RA 2nd, Phillips JJ, Douglas WH. Bond strength of six dentinal adhesives. J Dent 1994; 22:92–96
68. Versluis A, Tantbirojn D, Douglas WH. Why do shear bond tests pull out dentin? J Dent Res 1997; 76:1298–1307
69. Sano H, Shono T, Sonoda H, Takatsu T, Ciucchi B, Carvalho R, Pashley DH. Relationship between surface area for adhesion and tensile bond strength: evaluation of a micro-tensile bond test. Dent Mater 1994; 10:236–240
70. Pashley DH, Carvalho RM, Sano H, Nakajima M, Yoshiyama M, Shono Y, Fernandes CA, Tay F. The microtensile bond test: a review. J Adhes Dent 1999; 1:299–309
71. DeHoff PH, Anusavice KJ, Wang Z. Three-dimensional finite element analysis of the shear bond test. Dent Mater 1995; 11:126–131

Part III
Bonding to Cementum

Composition and Structure of Cementum: Strategies for Bonding

8

D. Tziafas

Introduction

The cervical margin of class-II and class-V cavities is usually located below the cemento-enamel junction. This area poses a clinical problem in adhesive resin restorations, since the margins of the cavities are limited by cementum (Fig. 8.1), a calcified tissue exhibiting several histo-morphological and functional variations from the dental structures that have been extensively evaluated as bonding substrates (enamel and dentin).

Cementum is a specialized connective tissue covering the outermost layer of calcified matrix on root surface, with a primary role to connect the periodontal ligament to the root surface. Cementum has not been largely encountered as a substrate from the bonding point of view, despite the fact that cervical microleakage has been early recognized to contribute to high incidence of secondary caries and

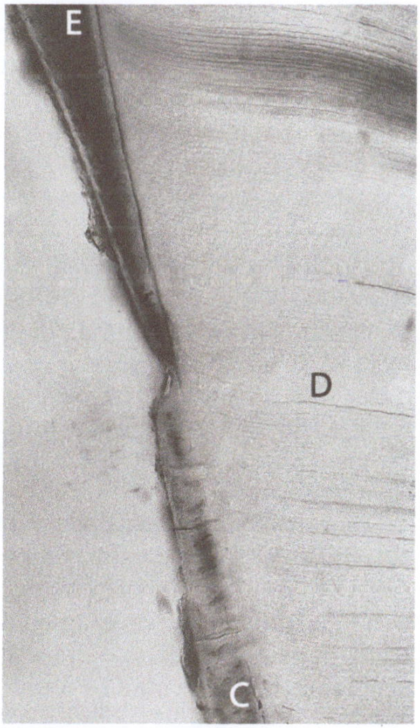

Fig. 8.1. Light micrograph of a ground section of an adult human canine. Enamel (*E*), dentin (*D*) and cementum (*C*) at cervical tooth situation

fail of restorations [1, 2]. Very few studies have evaluated cementum-bonding restorations and the techniques used in present clinical practice in terms of their effectiveness and predictability [2–6].

A systematic approach to bonding at the cervical margins of class-II and class-V restorations requires understanding of anatomy and histo-physiology of the root dental structures.

This chapter reviews the main structural, compositional, and functional aspects of cementum, and its primary evaluation as a bonding substrate.

Developmental and Structural Aspects

Cementum Varieties and Their Locations

Three varieties of cementum cover the root of the human tooth: acellular afibrillar cementum; acellular extrinsic fiber cementum, and cellular mixed-stratified cementum. Their location and structural characteristics are associated with their different functional identity [7–10].

Acellular afibrillar cementum. Acellular afibrillar cementum is located mainly around the cemento-enamel junction covering further small enamel areas. Its distribution pattern varies from tooth to tooth and along the cemento-enamel junction of the same tooth [9]. By light and electron microscopy acellular afibrillar cementum represents a non-homogenous matrix composed of multiple calcified layers without collagen fibers [11].

Acellular extrinsic fiber cementum. The acellular extrinsic fiber cementum constitutes the majority of the cementum. It represents a thin layer of mineralized tissue located along the coronal two-thirds of the root surface (Fig. 8.2 a, b). In anterior teeth acellular extrinsic fiber cementum is further extended to the apical root third. The formation of this type of cementum (Fig. 8.2 c) is a continuous process characterized by an extremely slow rate of new matrix deposition [12]; thus, it reaches a thickness of approximately 15 µm during the prefunctional stage of root development, and a total thickness of approximately 50 µm during the functional stage throughout the life of the tooth [13, 14]. The periodic deposition of this type of cementum is seen in light microscopy as multiple layers of matrix interspersed by growth lines.

Cellular mixed stratified cementum. Cellular mixed stratified cementum is composed of multiple interposed layers of acellular extrinsic fiber cementum and cellular intrinsic fiber cementum (Fig. 8.2 d, e), which is mainly deposited on the apical root surface area and in the furcation areas. In fact, pure cellular intrinsic fiber cementum is only deposited as a part of the reparative process following root resorption [15]. The appositional growth of cellular cementum is much faster that acellular cementum, reaching a mean thickness of more than 200 µm [16]. In adult teeth, impacted teeth, and in teeth without antagonists, extremely thick layers of cellular cementum could be found around the apical third of their roots [9, 17].

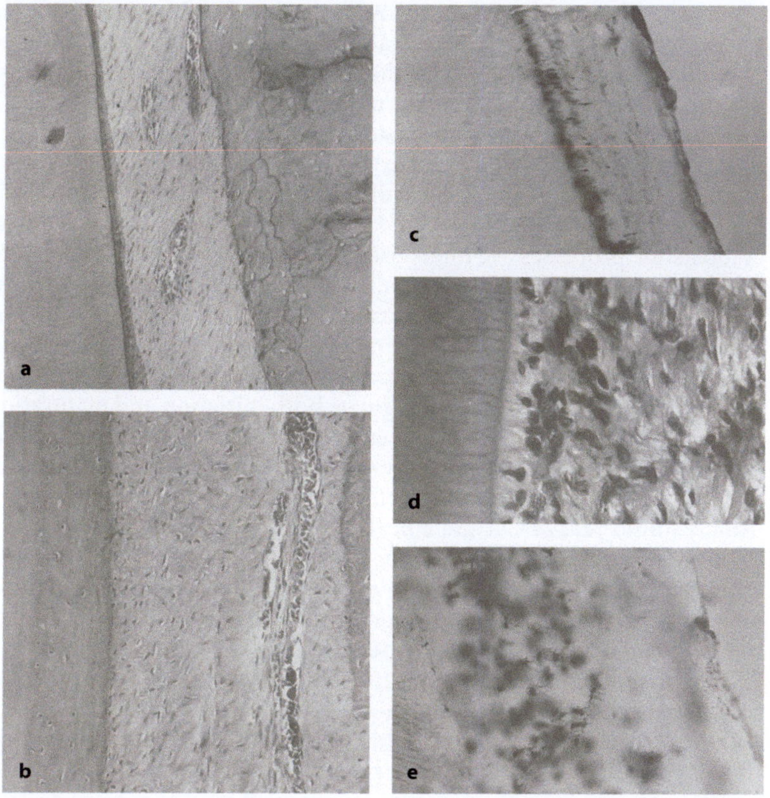

Fig. 8.2 a–e. Light micrographs of the main types of cementum. **a** Demineralized section of adult dog molar. Acellular extrinsic fiber cementum. **b** Ground section of adult human premolar. Acellular extrinsic fiber cementum. Note the dentino-cemental junction. **c** Demineralized section of developing dog molar. Cuboidal-shaped cementoblasts forming acellular extrinsic fiber cementum. **d** Apical situation from the section seen in **a**. Cellular mixed stratified cementum. **e** Apical situation from the section seen in **d**. Cellular mixed stratified cementum with numerous cementocyte lacunae

The primary role of acellular extrinsic fiber cementum is to attach periodontal ligament fibers to the root surface, supporting tooth mobility and function. Cellular cementum has important functional role in maintaining the occlusal relationship of the tooth and repairing the resorbed root surface areas. Furthermore, acellular afibrillar cementum seems to have only adaptive function.

Cementum Formation

Cellular and molecular mechanisms, which regulate formation of periodontal tissues, including cementum, have not been fully understood. It is well known that dental follicle cells of ectomesenchymal origin are capable of forming cementum when properly stimulated [18–20]. As to the nature of the cementum-forming cells (cementoblasts), there is a widely accepted opinion that they represent a population of periodontal cells [9, 21], although some authors suggest that epithelial cells may also contribute to the process of cementum formation [22–24].

The differentiation of dental follicle cells into cementoblasts is closely related to root dentin formation at a band extending 200–300 µm coronally to the developing root edge [9]. Progenitor cells migrate towards the newly deposited, but not yet mineralized, dentin matrix, as the Hertwig's root sheath breaks down. Numerous cytoplasmic processes are interposed between the dentinal collagen fibers, forming the dentino-cemental junction [14]. A layer of new matrix (precementum or cementoid) is deposited onto the external surface of the dentin by the surface root lining cells in a polar pattern. Recently, Nociti et al. [20] reported that the levels of inorganic pyrophosphate within the extracellular matrix of periodontal ligament is one of the crucial factors that regulate both initiation and maturation of cementum. Early mineralization of precementum into acellular extrinsic fiber cementum by deposition of hydroxyapatite crystals initially between and then within the collagen fibers, before the complete mineralization of the mantle root dentin, is usually found [25, 26]. At the apical third, highly active cementum-forming cells [12] deposit matrix in a non-polar bone-like pattern (cellular cementum). Cells entrapped into cellular cementum are called cementocytes. In mature teeth acellular cementum is not covered by precementum, a 3- to 5-µm-width layer which is usually seen along the cellular cementum [27, 28].

The formation of cementum is characterized by apposition throughout the functional stage of the tooth life. Since the collagen fibers of the periodontal ligament undergo remodeling, acellular cementum formation providing attachment to Sharpey's fibers is a continuous process. New cementoblasts seem to be continuously recruited from the periodontal ligament pool to replace destroyed cementoblasts or cementoblasts that have reached the end of their life span [9]; however, it is not generally agreed that a specialized cell type exists in the periodontal ligament for the continuous cementum formation. Whether cementoblasts-forming acellular extrinsic fiber cementum are phenotypically different from the periodontal fibroblasts, or further cementoblasts-forming cellular cementum are specific cells or "osteoblast variants," is still not known [30].

The root surface covered by the acellular extrinsic fiber cementum is an area at risk of carious demineralization or invasion by plaque bacteria. Regeneration of cervical dental structures is of clinical importance, and it seems challenging to devise new therapeutic methods enhancing cementum regeneration in affected root surfaces. More particularly, with regard to restorative strategies, novel biomaterials aiming to induce controlled formation of acellular extrinsic fiber cementum might be designed.

Structural Characteristics of Acellular Extrinsic Fiber Cementum

Acellular extrinsic fiber cementum is not a homogenously calcified tissue (Fig. 8.3). Cementum is characterized by amorphous mineralized microstructures and a dense network of unmineralized Sharpey's fibers, oriented perpendicularly to the root dentin. At the onset of cementum formation these fibers are extremely

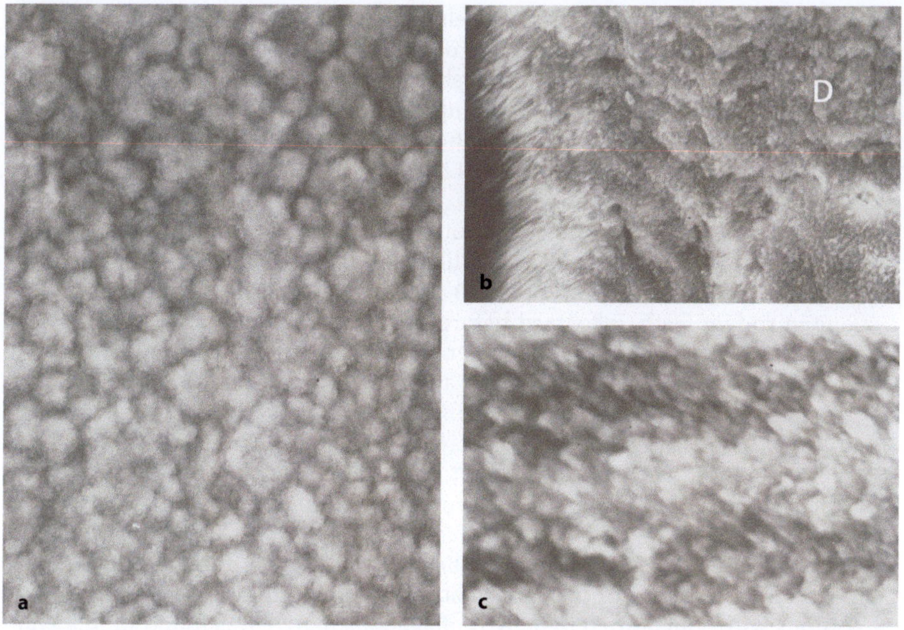

Fig. 8.3 a–c. Scanning electron micrographs of adult human acellular extrinsic fiber cementum at cervical tooth situation. **a** Root surface. The non-homogenously calcified structure of cementum. **b** Longitudinal section from the same root area. The uncalcified core of Sharpey's fiber oriented perpendicularly to the root dentin (*D*). **c** Higher magnification of **b**. Atypical organization of apatite crystals

short, whereas in mature teeth they are continuous with the long periodontal ligament fibers. These fiber types are clearly distinguishable from a small number of intrinsic collagen fibers, which are also found in acellular cementum. Hydroxyapatite crystals, perpendicularly deposited to the root surface, between or within the collagen fibers, form crystals of 1–4 µm in length over a long period of time [27, 31]. In light microscopy acellular extrinsic fiber cementum is characterized by the presence of incremental lines, oriented parallel to the root surface.

The Cemento-Enamel and Dentino-Cemental Junctions

The junction between cementum and enamel exhibits three normal variations:

1. Cementum overlaps the cervical border of enamel in more than 60% of the human teeth.
2. Cementum meets directly the enamel in approximately 30% of the human teeth.
3. In <10%, a gap (exposing the dentin surface) exists between enamel and cementum.

The dentino-cemental junction is developed as a result of the multiple events occurring during the early stages of root formation, i.e., root dentinogenesis, cementum formation, epithelial root sheath disorganization, and periodontal ligament formation. Cementum-forming cells differentiating along the newly deposited predentin produce collagen fibers which are integrated between the collagen fibers of the predentin matrix [12]. Two structures have been associated with the dentino-cemental junction:

1. The intermediate cementum. Some authors have reported the presence of a glycoprotein-rich matrix, or an enamel-like material at the interface between root dentin and cementum. This 10- to 20-μm-thick layer, characterized as hyaline zone in rodent teeth, is formed before cementum deposition, and it has been associated with cementum attachment to root dentin. Its existence in human teeth has been reported only for the apical portion of the root [32]. The presence of this collagen-free matrix at the junction between acellular cementum and root dentin and its origin is controversial [33, 34]. Thomas [12] stated that the junction is formed as a slow accretion of mineral on the root dentin surface, rather than the accumulation of minerals within a preformed collagenous matrix.
2. Tomes' granular layer. This layer has been described as a number of dark granules in the periphery of the root dentin underlying the cementum in ground sections with transmitted light. No collagenous matrix was found in this granular layer. Most authors believe that it represents a structure caused by the looping of the dentinal tubules in that region [35]. While peripheral dentin in the crown contains multiply branched dentinal tubules, the peripheral root dentin is atubular. Only in the subjacent granular area are dentinal tubules localized, but in a somewhat chaotic manner [36].

Biochemistry of Mature Cementum

Cementum represents the less characterized mineralized tissue. Similarly to the other connective calcified tissues, approximately 40% of extracellular organic matrix and 50–60% of hydroxyapatite crystals are composed of water [35]. In general, the two major types of cementum (acellular extrinsic fiber cementum and cellular mixed stratified cementum) are similar to bone, with three crucial exceptions:

1. Cementum is avascular.
2. Since cementoblasts do not express parathormone receptors (as do osteoblasts), cementum does not undergo remodeling [37].
3. Tissue-specific proteins have been identified in the cementum [38, 39].

Extracellular Matrix

The extracellular matrix of human cementum consists mainly of collagen type I (90% of the organic matrix) and collagen type III (5%) according to the classic study by Cristoffersen and Landis [40]. In all connective tissues collagen molecules play important structural roles, providing the functional tissue scaffold.

Furthermore, a number of non-collagenous cell attachment proteins, with only partially characterized properties, have been detected in cementum [29]:

1. Fibronectin, osteopontin, and osteocalcin with possible role in cementum development and regeneration.
2. Vitronectin, an adhesion molecule found in high concentration in serum with unknown function.
3. Cementum attachment protein (and possibly other yet unidentified adhesion molecules) and cementum growth factor are tissue-specific molecules, although some homology to known bone proteins has been reported [38, 39]. Cementum attachment protein binds with fibronectin and hydroxyapatite but not with collagen [41]. It supports the attachment of mesenchymal cells, but not of epithelial cells [41].
4. Enamel proteins have been detected in cementoblasts, but their presence in cementum extracellular matrix has not yet been demonstrated [9].
5. Alkaline phosphatase, playing a role in precipitation of calcium phosphate salts, is at least partially found in a collagen-bound form [42].

Inorganic Component

The inorganic component of cementum is the same as in other calcified tissues, bone, dentin, and enamel. Chemical analysis of the cementum inorganic phase has shown that the primary mineral component is hydroxyapatite $[Ca_{10}(PO_4)_6(OH)_2]$ containing amounts of amorphous calcium phosphate. In transmission electron micrographs hydroxyapatite crystals are found mainly between the collagen fibrils, normally arranged with their c-axis parallel to the long axis of collagen fibrils [27].

The crystallinity of the cemental inorganic component is lower than the other calcified tissues [9]. As a result, cementum is decalcified more easily, while it has a greater affinity for adsorption of environmental ions (i.e., fluoride). In general, cementum of adult mature teeth has a higher fluoride content in comparison with the other calcified tissues [43–45]. The Mg content in cementum is about half that in dentin. There is a gradual increase of Mg present in the cementum from periphery to deeper layers [43, 46]. Trace elemental concentrations of Cu, Zn, and Na were further detected by electron microprobe analysis in human root cementum of healthy and periodontally involved teeth [47].

Cementum in Health and Disease

Root Permeability

The physiology of root-calcified tissue system has not been studied systematically. With regard to permeability of cementum in health and disease, contrary data have been reported. In general, the cemental matrix is porous allowing only permeation of water and inorganic ions under physiological tissue conditions. Nevertheless, the structure of diseased root surface is also permeable to saliva organic components and plaque bacterial byproducts.

In periodontally involved teeth, plaque bacterial products have been detected in the 10- to 12-µm-deep surface layer [48]. Furthermore, Lygre et al. [49] found bacterial lipopolysaccharide at a distance of 70 µm from the surface of the periodontally diseased roots. Penetration of substances derived from saliva to the exposed root cementum might be attributed mainly to numerous cracks and fractures, which are developed at the non-supported areas with cells and fiber root surface [9]. Invasion of bacteria into cemental matrix has been demonstrated in chronic periodontal pathosis [48, 50]. Infected cementum has been characterized as a reservoir of periodontopathogenic bacteria [50].

In teeth with heavily infected root canals bacterial substances have been detected near the dentino-cemental junction [51]. In an experimental study, necrosis of cementocytes was found after root canal treatment in rat molar teeth [52].

Age Changes in Cementum

Cementum grows appositionally throughout life at a linear rate [53], although the variations in width of incremental lines indicate that the rate of cementum deposition varies from period to period. Generally, cementum increases in thickness by different growth patterns among types of cementum being formed. Its thickness varies greatly with tooth group, tooth surface area, and cervical/apical root positions [54]. Cementum, like bone, is a dynamic tissue, capable of responding to occlusal forces and physiological tooth movement. The greatest amount of cementum is deposited apically, constricting the apical foramen, and in the furcations of multi-rooted teeth. According to Schroeder [7], cementum is thicker in areas exposed to tensional forces, whereas Dastmalchi et al. [55] found that cementum thickness is increased more rapidly at the distal than the mesial parts of root surface.

Root Surface Caries and Cementum

The increased number of teeth in older individuals, due to caries preventive strategies, resulted in higher prevalence of root caries during the past two decades. Root caries occurs on exposed tooth surfaces below the cemento-enamel junction after gingival recession. Cariogenic plaque, rather than periodontitis or gingival inflammation, is the essential factor responsible for root caries development. The different forms of root surface caries, ranging from minor undemineralized and discolored areas to extensive yellow-brown soft areas, are rarely associated with cavitation below the affected cementum [56, 57].

The histopathology of root caries is similar to that of enamel carious lesions. The early root caries lesion appears as a zone of demineralization deep to the root surface. The radiolucent area is usually detected below a well-mineralized layer of acellular extrinsic fiber cementum, which varies in thickness and mineral contents. Nyvad et al. [58] described in an experimentally induced root caries model the initial histopathological changes seen after covering of exposed cementum with plaque. Within 1–3 months a continuous subsurface loss of mineral was associated with redeposition of minerals in the surface cementum layer which appeared hypermineralized when compared with the neighboring cementum. Larger apatite crystals were found in the root surface of the caries-affected cementum [59]. Bacteria infiltrating the lesion split the collagen fibers of the cementum and were frequently detected at the dentino-cementum junction [60, 61]. Bacteria were also identified within the subjacent dentinal tubules during early root caries development [62]. As in enamel, caries active and arrested or slowly progressive lesions may be seen in cementum. Active root surface lesion presents a well-defined area of softening and yellowish discoloration. Inactive root surface lesion appears hard on probing with dark discoloration. Transitory stages between active and arrested root surface caries cannot be excluded.

Changes of Cementum in Periodontally Involved Teeth

In periodontally involved teeth, the exposure of acellular extrinsic fiber cementum to the environment of oral cavity or periodontal pocket creates constantly changes in the surface structure and composition of cemental matrix and eventually diseases of the root calcified tissues, such as development of cementum caries and cervical root resorption.

Structural modifications of the cementum surface are characterized mainly by loss of collagen cross-banding, breakdown of dentogingival fibers, and dissolution of mineral components [63, 64]. Bosshardt and Selvig [9] state that these surface-limited modifications transitionally extent to the subsurface tissue area and can be described only by electron microscopy. It has been reported that surface fractures and cracks are also developed at the exposed cementum.

It has been repeatedly demonstrated by chemical [45, 66], microradiographic [58, 64, 67, 68], and SEM-microprobe [43] investigations that the exposed cementum surface is progressively hypermineralized, although Barton and Van Swol [47] and Cohen et al. [69] did not detect such a hypermineralized zone. Furseth [70] found that this zone can be experimentally created 21 days after a gingivectomy procedure, whereas it can be re-established 4–8 weeks after removal of the hypermineralized cementum surface by root planning [64]. The cementum hypermineralization is related to the loss of cross-banding after chronic exposure of root surface to the oral environment [43, 71]. Atypical development and orientation of large apatite crystals characterize the surface structure of hypermineralized cementum in an SEM. The atypical distribution of mineral components and the increased fluoride concentration in this zone may explain the resistance of hypermineralized cementum to acid demineralization [68].

In periodontally involved teeth, especially in cases of hyperplastic gingivitis, large resorptive defects in the cervical region of vital teeth are usually found. This phenomenon is called cervical root resorption or idiopathic root resorption, and its nature has not been adequately elucidated [37, 72]. The defect penetrates deep into the tooth, and areas of the dentin are replaced by formation of inflamed soft tissue and defective hard tissue of periodontal origin. This type of resorption is usually prevented by the downgrowth of cervical epithelium [73]. External root resorption associated with periodontal trauma has been distinguished by Andreasen [74] into the surface resorption, inflammatory resorption, and replacement resorption (ankylosis). Two structural components of cementum have been related to prevention of external root resorption; the layer of cementoblasts and the zone of precementum. Damage of cementoblasts combined with absence of precementum zone is considered to cause initiation of the resorptive process.

Strategies for Bonding to Root Dental Structures

D. Tziafas, G. Eliades

One of the most frequent clinical problems associated with class-II and class-V cavities in adhesive resin restorations is the weak link of restorative material to root dental structures, when the cervical margin is located below the cemento-enamel junction. In terms of cementum, the tissue-bonding properties have not been adequately elucidated.

The Problem

Most studies on adhesive bonding to root surfaces deal with the bonding mechanism of adhesive systems to exposed cervical dentin surfaces (sound, sclerotic, or carious) [75, 76], without giving particular attention to cementum. Nevertheless, cementum usually occupies the critical cervical marginal edge of the complex cervical restorations extending beyond the cementum-enamel junction. Moreover, it is implicated in the adhesive treatment of cervical hypersensitivity of newly exposed root surfaces after periodontal scaling.

Since complete cementum removal is not considered a realistic approach in periodontal therapy [77], desensitizing agents based on dental-adhesive technology are frequently used for pain relief. It is well known that root surfaces exposed for a long period to the oral environment develop a superficial hypermineralized layer with limited permeability, compared with intact cementum. These surfaces may interfere in the marginal quality of root restorations, especially in elderly population.

Very limited information exists on cementum-bonded restorations [2–6, 74]. Ferrari et al. [5] reported that cementum treated with dentin bonding systems is infiltrated by the resin, but the predictability of the bond is unclear. Van Dijken et al. [78] found excellent adaptation in the cervical margins located below the cemento-enamel junction with the directed shrinkage technique; however, in vitro measurements evaluating similar restorative techniques have shown moderate to severe leakage in cementum, with almost no leakage in enamel [2, 6]. Recent studies evaluating the bond strength of restorative materials to the three calcified dental tissues put important questions about the contribution of cervically bonded materials to the mechanical properties of restorations [5, 79, 80]. Such controversial findings show that our knowledge on bonding to cementum is limited. Furthermore, it is still unclear whether or not the problem of bonding to cementum is related to the structure and properties of the tissue or to a limited effectiveness of the adhesive materials at the region.

Treatment of intact and periodontitis-affected cementum with acidic (citric acid of pH:1, 37% phosphoric acid of pH:1) and neutral (24% EDTA·2NaOH of pH:7) conditioners revealed a higher demineralization capacity of the EDTA solution on both substrates; however, the morphology of the periodontitis-affected cementum surface was highly variable, with islands of dense granular material [81]. Based on these findings, mechanical removal of the superficial layer of the exposed cementum prior to any periodontal regenerative treatment has been advised. This treatment mode may be applied to improve adhesive bonding as well.

From a surface science perspective, intact cementum demonstrates a completely different composition from smear-layer covered dentin, the latter being the most common substrate for adhesive bonding. X-ray photoelectron spectroscopy showed a strong reduction in the Ca/C ratio of intact cementum surfaces compared with smear-layer covered dentin surfaces (0.07 vs 0.43); however, the apatitic structure of the inorganic phase was more preserved in cementum surfaces (Ca/P ratio 1.69 vs 1.13), being close to the theoretical hydroxyapatite value (Fig. 8.4a, b) [82, 83]. These results imply that organic material predominates on the outmost cementum surface. Treatment of intact cementum surface with 17% EDTA·4NaOH (pH:7.4) further reduced the Ca/C (0.05) and the Ca/P (1.08) ratios due to demineralization. The shear bond strength of a resin composite to EDTA conditioned sound cementum, after treatment with an aqueous primer composed of 5% glutaraldehyde and 35% hydroxyethyl methacrylate, was estimated as 6 MPa, a value statistically significantly lower than the corresponding value for dentin [82, 83]. It seems that after demineralization the increased intrinsic fibrial content of intact cementum surface creates an organic network that lacks the cohesive strength of demineralized dentin collagen, and although it is reinforced by resin infiltration [5], results in low bond strength. From the variety of the dental adhesive systems currently available (three step, two step, self-etching), the traditional three-step multicomponent adhesives provided surface and interfacial characteristics of intact cementum more compatible with conventional dentin hybridization [84].

Treatment of cervical hypersensitivity with general-purpose hydrophilic dental adhesives or specially designed polymerizable sealers is one of the in-office methods available, aiming to reduce tissue permeability and/or nerve excitation capacity. Based on the hydrodynamic theory of pain perception in dentin [85] and the in vivo dentin biopsy studies from hypersensitive and non-sensitive areas [86, 87], the extent of dental tubule occlusion and the reduction in dentin hydraulic conductance are considered as the two major treatment requirements that have been used as well for the in vitro screening of the effectiveness of desensitizing agents [88]; however, no clear relationship was found in vitro between extent of tubule occlusion and hydraulic conductance analysis [88, 89]. Moreover, clinically effective agents failed to meet these criteria, indicating that other mechanisms may contribute as well. The role of residual cementum thickness, especially in the treatment of post-scaling sensitivity, is unknown. Some of the polymerizable desensitizing sealers contain biological fixatives, crosslinking agents, and hydrogels that may react with proteins or other extracellular components. The contribution of the intrinsic cementum fibrial network to the nucleation of such reactions has not been investigated. Treatment of these surfaces with glass ionomer liners seems problematic. The minimal film thickness, viscosity, and surface tension requirements for desensitization treatments without cervical tissue loss do not allow for placement of glass ionomer liners, without changing the anatomical form of the

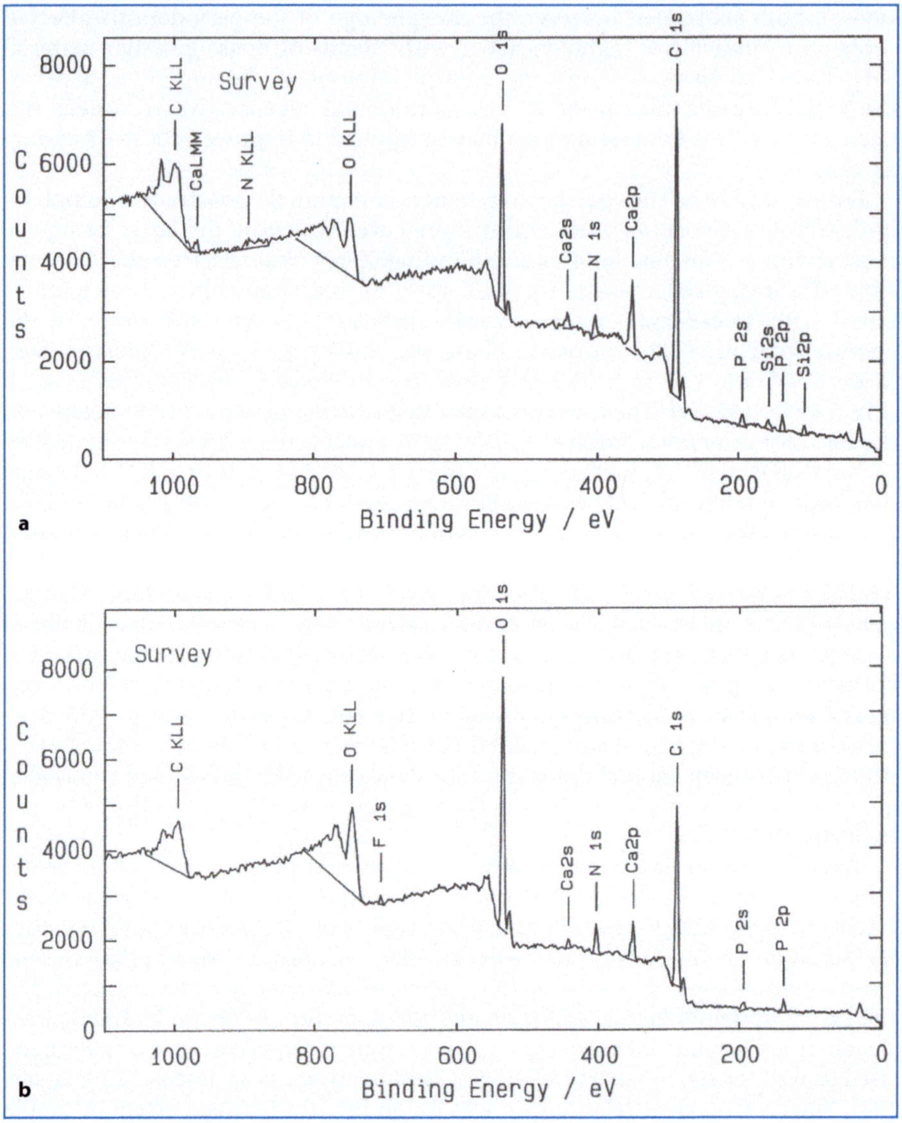

Fig. 8.4 a, b. X-ray photoelectron spectroscopy spectra of intact cementum before (**a**) and after (**b**) 20 s conditioning with 17% EDTA·4NaOH (pH:7.4) aqueous solution. Note the presence of fluorine on conditioned surface

region. Also, the presence of the fibrial arrangement may provide a diffusion barrier to the inorganic phase for adequate sealing.

Hypermineralized cementum, after long-term intraoral exposure, may appear as the most suitable substrate for the strong ionic reactivity of glass ionomers with mineralized tissues and capacity for molecular bond formation; however, poor marginal integrity at the cervical matrix is a common clinical finding in conventional glass ionomers. This is considered to be the result of the low flexural fatigue limit of these brittle materials, which buffer the tensile stresses developed at the cervical region during functional loading, and by marginal deterioration prevents bulk fractures or debonding [90]. Resin-modified glass ionomer processing improved flexural fatigue limits and hybrid layer formation with conditioned or primed cavity walls, demonstrating marginal discrepancies as well, which possibly developed after a short post-insertion period [91].

Future Directions

Modification of intact cementum surfaces to improve adhesion may include a eproteination step, prior to any adhesive treatment, in order to remove the high organic content and expose the inorganic substrate, like conditioning with aqueous solutions of sodium hypochlorite (NaOCl).

NaOCl is a well-known, non-specific proteolytic agent that demonstrates effective removal of organic constituents from biological materials at room temperature. The proteolytic action of NaOCl involves extensive fragmentation of long peptide chains and formation of n-chloramines with terminal amine groups that may form other byproducts, including inter- and intramolecular crosslinks via Schiff base formation [92]. NaOCl has been advocated as an intermediate conditioning treatment of acid-demineralized dentin, in order to remove exposed collagen and produce protein-depleted channels into subsurface intact dentin for resin diffusion, thus creating the so-called reverse hybrid layer [93]. Such dentin surfaces have been proposed as mineralized, hydrophilic alternatives to collagen-rich, hydrophobic acid-demineralized dentin, possessing increased stiffness and stability to degradation [94]. Since the intrinsic fibrial arrangement of intact cementum is not calcified, the deproteination capacity of NaOCl may be intensified by employing a rubbing action. Freshly prepared 10% solutions may efficiently remove the fibrial arrangement within a time period of conventional conditioning treatments (i.e., 20 s).

Low-energy laser treatment may be used as well for removal of the intrinsic fibrial arrangement of cementum; however, no information exists on such applications. Laser irradiation under the conditions used for treatment of dentin hypersensitivity (fusion of exposed dentin tubules) may alter the structure and composition of the substrate towards a non-compatible surface for currently available adhesive systems.

As the patterns of oral disease continue to evolve, restorative strategies in future research will include the root-calcified tissue system. A complete understanding of tissue microstructure and chemical composition and the basic reaction patterns of root dentin and cementum to restorative techniques and materials must be pursued. In addition to the future directions in adhesive dentistry [95], advances in biotechnology, such as the biomimetic molecular-based applications, might not be excluded from the designing of novel biomaterials. It always must be remembered that the cervical margin of restorations located below the cemento-enamel junction is primarily an area of vital tissue therapy.

References

1. Mjör IA. The location of clinically diagnosed secondary caries. Ouintessence Int 1988; 29:313–317
2. Beznos C. Microleakage at the cervical margin of composite class II cavities with different restorative techniques. Oper Dent 2001; 26:60–69
3. Hargraves JA, Grossman ES, Matejka JM. Scanning electron microscopic study of prepared cavities involving enamel, dentin and cementum. J Prosth Dent 1989; 61:191–197
4. Tay FR, Gwinnett AJ, Pang KM, Wei SHY. Variability in microleakage observed in a total-etch wet-bonding technique under different handling conditions. J Dent Res 1995; 74:1168–1178
5. Ferrari M, Cagidiago MC, Davidson C. Resistance of cementum in class II and V cavities to penetration by an adhesive system. Dent Mater 1997; 13:157–162
6. Demarco FF, Ramos OLV, Mota CS, Formolo E, Justino LM. Influence of different restorative techniques on microleakage in class II cavities with gingival wall in cementum. Oper Dent 2001; 26:253–259
7. Schroeder UE. Oral structural biology. Thieme, Zurich, 1991
8. Avery JK. Oral development and histology, 2nd edn. Thieme, New York, 1994
9. Bosshardt DD, Selvig KA. Dental cementum: the dynamic tissue covering of the root. Periodontology 1997; 13:41–75
10. ten Cate AR. Oral histology. Development, structure and function, 5th edn. Mosby, St. Louis, 1998
11. Beertsen W, Van den Bos T. Alkaline phosphatase induces the deposition of calcified layers in relation to dentin: an in vitro study to mimic the formation of afibrillar acellular cementum. J Dent Res 1990; 69:1669–1673
12. Thomas HF. Root formation. Int J Devel Biol 1995; 39:231–237
13. Bosshardt DD, Schroeder HE. Establishment of acellular extrinsic fiber cementum on human teeth. A light- and electron-microscopic study. Cell Tissue Res 1991; 263:325–336
14. Bosshardt DD, Schroeder HE. Cementogenesis reviewed: a comparison between human premolars and rodent molars. Anat Rec 1996; 245:267–292
15. Schroeder HE. Human cellular mixed stratified cementum: a tissue with alternating layers of acellular extrinsic and cellular intrinsic fiber cementum. Schweiz Monatsschr Zahned 1993; 103:550–560
16. Schroeder HE. Biological problems of regenerative cementogenesis: synthesis and attachment of collagenous matrices on growing and established root surfaces. Int Rev Cytol 1992; 142:1–59
17. Azaz B, Ulmansky M, Moshev R, Sela J. Correlation between age and thickness of cementum in impacted teeth. Oral Surg Oral Med Oral Pathol 1974; 38:691–694
18. ten Cate AR, Mills C. The development of the periodontium: the origin of alveolar bone. Anat Rec 1972; 173:69–78
19. Palmer RM, Lumsden AS. Development of periodontal ligament and alveolar bone in homografted recombinations of enamel organs and papillary, pulpal and follicular mesenchyme in the mouse. Arch Oral Biol 1987; 32:281–289
20. Nociti FH, Berry JE, Foster BL, Gurley KA, Kingsley DM, Takata T, Miyaushi M, Somerman MJ. Cementum: a phosphate sensitive tissue. J Dent Res 2002; 81:817–821
21. Beertsen W, Van den Bos T, Everts V. Continuous growth of acellular extrinsic fiber cementum. A review. Acta Med Dent Helv 1997; 2:103–115
22. Slavkin HC, Boyde A. Cementum: an epithelial secretory product? J Dent Res 1974; 53:157
23. MacNeil RL, Thomas HF. Development of the murine periodontium. I. Role of basement membrane in formation of a mineralized tissue on the developing root dentin surface. J Periodontol 1993; 64:95–102
24. Hammarstrom L, Alatli I, Fong CD. Origins of cementum. Oral Dis 1996; 2:63–69
25. Heritier M. Experimental induction of cementogenesis on the enamel of transplanted mouse tooth germs. Arch Oral Biol 1982; 27:87–97

26. Yamamoto H, Masuda, Toeda K, Suzuki K. Microradiographic and histopathological study of the cementum. Bull Tokyo Med Dent Univ 1962; 9:141–150
27. Selvig KA. The fine structure of human cementum. Acta Odontol Scand 1965; 23:423–441
28. Furseth R, Johansen E. A microradiographic comparison of sound and carious human dental cementum. Arch Oral Biol 1968; 13:1197–1206
29. MacNeil RL, D'Errico JA, Ouyang H, Berry J, Strayhorn C, Somerman MJ. Isolation of murine cementoblasts: unique cells or uniquely positioned osteoblasts? Eur J Oral Sci 1998 (Suppl I):350–356
30. Bar Kana I, Savion N, Narayanan AS, Pittaru S. Cementum attachment protein manifestation is restricted to the mineralized tissue forming cells of the periodontium. Eur J Oral Sci 1998 (Suppl I):357–364
31. Yamamoto T. The innermost layer of cementum in rat molars: its ultrastucture, development, and calcification. Arch Histol Jpn 1986; 49:459–481
32. Bencze L. Befunde an der Dentinzementgrenze. Stomatologie 1927; 5:887–896
33. Owens PDA. A light and electron microscopic study of the early stages of root surface formation in molar teeth in the rat. Arch Oral Biol 1980; 24:901–907
34. Yamamoto T, Wakita M. The development and structure of principal fibers and cellular cementum in rat molars. J Periodont Res 1991; 26:129–137
35. Davis WL. Oral histology. Cell structure and function. Saunders, Philadelphia, 1986
36. Weber DF. An improved technique for producing casts of the internal structure of hard tissues, including some observations on human dentine. Arch Oral Biol 1983; 28:885–891
37. Hammarstrom L, Lindskog S. Factors regulating and modifying dental root resorption. Proc Finn Dent Soc 1992; 88 (Suppl I):115–123
38. Yonemura K. Narayanan AS, Miki Y, Page RC, Okada H. Isolation and partial characterization of a growth factor from human cementum. Bone Miner 1992; 18:187–198
39. Wu D, Ikezawa K, Parker T, Saito M, Narayanan AS. Characterization of a collagenous cementum-derived attachment protein. J Bone Min Res 1996; 11:686–692
40. Christoffersen J, Landis WJ. A contribution with review to the description of mineralization of bone and other calcified tissues in vivo. Anat Rec 1991; 230:435–450
41. Pitaru S, Narayanan SA, Olson S, Savion N, Hekmati H, Alt I, Metzger Z. Specific cementum attachment protein enhances selectively the attachment and migration of periodontal cells to root surfaces. J Periodont Res 1995; 30:360–368
42. Groeneveld MC, Everts V, Beertsen W. Alkaline phosphatase activity in the periodontal ligament and gingiva of the rat molar: its relation to cementum formation. J Dent Res 1955; 74:1374–1381
43. Hals E, Selvig KA Correlated electron probe microanalysis and microradiography of carious and normal dental cementum. Caries Res 1977; 11:62–65
44. Weatherell JA, Robinson C. Fluoride in teeth and bone. In: Ekstrand J, Fejerskov O, Silvestone LM, eds. Fluoride in dentistry. Munksgaard, Copenhagen, 1988, pp 28–59
45. Nakata TM, Stepnick RJ, Zipkin I. Chemistry of human dental cementum: the effect of age and fluoride exposure on the concentration of ash, fluoride, calcium, phosphorus and magnesium. J Periodontol 1972; 43:115–124
46. Neiders ME, Eick JD, Miller WA, Leitner JW. Electron probe microanalysis of cementum and underlying dentin in young permanent teeth. J Dent Res 1972; 51:122–130
47. Barton NS, Van Swol RL. Periodontally diseased vs normal roots as evaluated by scanning electron microscopy and electron probe analysis. J Periodontol 1987; 58:634–638
48. Daly CG, Kieser JB, Corbet EF. Histological assessment of periodontally involved cementum. J Clin Periodontol 1982; 9:266–274
49. Lygre H, Solheim E, Gjerdet NR, Skaug N. Fatty acids of healthy and periodontally diseased root substance in human teeth. J Dent Res 1992; 71:43–46
50. Andriaens PA, De Boever JA, Loesche WJ. Bacterial invasion in root cementum and radicular dentin of periodontally diseased teeth in humans: a reservoir of periodontopathogenic bacteria. J Periodontol 1988; 59:222–230
51. Armitage GC, Christie TM. Structural changes in exposed human cementum. I. Light microscopic observations. J Periodont Res 1973; 8:343–355

52. Erasquin J, Muruzabal M. Necrosis of cementum induced by root canal treatments in the molar teeth of rats. Arch Oral Biol 1967; 12:1123–1132
53. Zander HA, hurzeler B. Continuous cementum apposition. J Dent Res 1958; 37:1035–1044
54. Bosshardt DD. Morphologische, morphodynamische und autoradiographische untersuchung der zementogenese an menschlichen zahnen. Thesis, Verlag Dr. Kovac, Hamburg, 1993
55. Dastmalchi R, Polson A, Bouwsma O, Proskin H. Cementum thickness and mesial drift. J Clin Periodontol 1990:17:709–713
56. Furseth R. A microradiographic and electron microscopic study of the cementum of human deciduous teeth. Acta Odontol Scand 1967; 25:613–645
57. Furseth R. The fine structure of the cellular cementum of young human teeth. Arch Oral Biol 1969; 14:1147–1158
58. Nyvad B, ten Cate JM, Fejerskov O. Microradiography of experimental root surface caries in man. Caries Res 1989; 23:218–223
59. Tohda H, Fejerskov O, Yanagisawa T. Transmission electron microscopy of cementum crystals correlated with Ca and F distribution in normal and carious human root surfaces. J Dent Res 1996; 75:949–954
60. Nyvad B, Fejerskov O. Active and inactive root surface caries: structural entites? In: Thylstrup A, Leach SA, Qvist V, eds. Dentine and dentine reactions in the oral cavity. IRL Press, Oxford, 1987
61. Nyvad B, Fejerskov O. An ultrastructural study of bacteria invasion and tissue breakdown in human experimental root surface caries. J Dent Res 1990; 69:2218–2225
62. Kidd EAM, Joyston-Bechal S. Essentials of dental caries. The disease and its management. Oxford University Press, New York, 1995
63. Selvig KA. Nonbanded fibrils of collagenous nature in human periodontal connective tissue. J Periodont Res 1968; 3:169–179
64. Selvig KA. Biological changes at the tooth–saliva interface in periodontal disease. J Dent Res 1969; 48:846–855
65. Nakib NM, Bissada NF, Simmelink JW, Goldstine SN. Endotoxin penetration into cementum of periodontally healthy and diseased human teeth. J Periodontol 1982; 53:368–378
66. Wirthlin ME, Pedersen ED, Hancock EB, Lamberts BL, Leonard EP. The hypermineralization of diseased root surfaces. J Periodontol 1979; 50:125–127
67. Yamamoto H, Sugahara N, Yamada N. Histopathological and microradiographic study of the exposed cementum from periodontally diseased human teeth. Bull Tokyo Med Dent Univ 1966; 13:407–421
68. Furseth R. Further observations on the fine structure of orally exposed and carious human dental cementum. Arch Oral Biol 1971; 16:71–85
69. Cohen M, Garnick JJ, Ringle RD, Hanes PJ, Thompson WO. Calcium and phosphorus content of roots exposed to the oral environment. J Clin Periodontol 1992; 9:268–273
70. Furseth R. A study of experimentally exposed and fluoride treated dental cementum in pigs. Acta Odontol Scand 1970; 28:833–850
71. Yamada N. Fine structure of exposed cementum in periodontal disease. Bull Tokyo Med Dent Univ 1968; 15:409–434
72. Moody AB, Speculand B, Smith AJ, Basu MK. Muliple idiopathic external resorption of teeth. Intern J Oral Maxillofac Surg 1990; 19:200–202
73. Brosjo M, Anderssen K, Berg J-O, Lindskog S. An experimental model for cervical resorption in monkeys. Endod Dent Traumatol 1990; 6:118–120
74. Andreasen JO. Luxation injuries. In: Traumatic injuries of the teeth. Munksgaard, Copenhagen, 1981
75. Tay FR, Kwong SM, Itthagarun A, King NM, Yip HK, Moulding KM, Pashley DH. Bonding of a self-etching primer to noncarious cervical sclerotic dentin: interfacial ultrastructure and microtensile bond strength evaluation. J Adhesive Dent 2000; 2:9–28
76. Nakajima M, Sano H, Burrow MF, Tagami J, Yoshiyama M, Ebisu S, Ciucchi B, Russell CM, Pashley DH. Tensile bond strength and SEM evaluation of caries affected dentin using dentin adhesives. J Dent Res 1995; 74:1679–1688

77. O'Leary TJ, Kafrawy AH. Total cementum removal: a realistic objective? J Periodontol 1983; 54:221–226
78. Van Dijiken JWV, Horsted TP, Waern R. Directed polymerization shrinkage versus a horizontal incremental technique: interfacial adaptation in vivo in class II cavities. Amer J Dent 1998; 11:165–172
79. Abade PF, Bertacchini M, Polack A, Macchi RL. Adhesion of a compomer to dental structures. Quintessence Int 1997; 28:509–512
80. Cagitiaco MC, Ferrari M, Vichi, Davidson CL. Mapping of tubule and intertubule surface areas available for bonding in class V and class II preparations. J Dent 1997; 25:379–389
81. Blomlöf J. Root cementum appearance in healthy monkeys and periodontitis-prone patients after different etching modalities. J Clin Periodontol 1996; 23:12–18
82. Eliades G, Palaghias G, Vougiouklakis G. Bonding composites to cementum by Gluma: surface characterization and bond strength. J Dent Res 1991; 70:383, Abstract 940
83. Eliades G, Palaghias G, Vougiouklakis G. Surface reactions of adhesives on dentin. Dent Mater 1990; 6:208–216
84. Mountouris G, Eliades G. Effect of dental adhesives on cervical root cementum. Odontostom Proodos 2002; 56:448–460
85. Brännström M, Garberoglio R. The dentinal tubules and the odontoblast processes. Acta Odont Scand 1972; 30:291–311
86. Yoshiyama M, Masada J, Uchida A, Ishida H. Scanning electron microscopic characterization of sensitive vs insensitive human radicular dentin. J Dent Res 1989; 68:1498–1502
87. Yoshiyama M, Noiri Y, Ozaki K, Uchida A, Ishikawa Y, Ishida H. Transmission electron microscopic characterization of hypersensitive human radicular dentin. J Dent Res 1990; 1293–1297
88. Kolker JL, Vargas M, Armstrong SR, Dawson D. Effect of desensitizing agents on dentin permeability and dentin tubule occlusion. J Adhesive Dent 2002; 4:211–221
89. Zhang Y, Agee K, Pashley DH, Pashley EL. The effects of pain-free desensitizer on dentine permeability and tubule occlusion over time, in vitro. J Clin Periodontol 1998; 25:884–891
90. Kakaboura A. Aging of glass-ionomer cements. In: Eliades G, Eliades T, Brantley WA, Watts DC, eds. Dental materials in vivo, aging and related phenomena. Quintessence, Carol Stream, Illinois, pp 79–98
91. Ferrari M, Davidson CL. Sealing capacity of a resin-modified glass-ionomer and resin composite placed in vivo in class V restorations. Oper Dent 1996; 21:69–72
92. Hawkins CL, Davies MJ. Hypochlorite-induced damage to proteins: formation of nitrogen-centered radicals from lysine residues and their role in protein fragmentation. Biochem J 1998; 332:617–625
93. Prati C, Chersoni S, Pashley DH. Effect of removal of surface collagen fibrils on resin-dentin bonding. Dent Mater 1999; 15:123–331
94. Perdigão J, Thompson JY, Toledano M, Osorio R. An ultra morphological characterization of collagen-depleted etched dentin. Am J Dent 1999; 12:250–255
95. Tay FR, Pashley DH. Dental adhesives of the future. J Adhesive Dent 2002; 4:91–103

Subject Index

I

K

L

M

N

O

P

Q

R

S

T

U

V

W

Z

MIX
Papier aus verantwortungsvollen Quellen
Paper from responsible sources
FSC® C105338

If you have any concerns about our products,
you can contact us on
ProductSafety@springernature.com

In case Publisher is established outside the EU,
the EU authorized representative is:
Springer Nature Customer Service Center GmbH
Europaplatz 3, 69115 Heidelberg, Germany

Printed by Libri Plureos GmbH
in Hamburg, Germany